Can STRESS HEAL?

KENNETH H. COOPER, M.D.

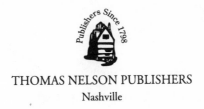

THOMAS NELSON PUBLISHERS

Nashville

Published in Nashville, Tennessee, by Thomas Nelson, Inc.,
Publishers.

The Bible version used in this publication is THE NEW KING
JAMES VERSION. Copyright © 1979, 1980, 1982, 1990,
Thomas Nelson, Inc., Publishers.

Library of Congress Cataloging-in-Publication Data

Cooper, Kenneth H.
    Can stress heal? : converting a major health hazard into
a surprising health benefit / Kenneth H. Cooper.
        p.   cm.
    Includes index.
    ISBN 0-7852-8315-3
    1. Stress management. 2. Stress (Physiology) 3. Stress
(Psychology) I. Title.
RA785.C66   1997
155.9'042—dc21   97-33082
                                                              CIP

Printed in the United States of America.

1 2 3 4 5 6 BVG 02 01 00 99 98 97

To the greatest answer to stress that a man could have—my family. Their support, prayers, advice, and calming presence have enabled me to discover the ultimate paradox: It is actually possible to experience joy in stress.

Contents

Acknowledgments

A book on the latest research findings and treatment techniques for stress must, by its very nature, be a work in progress. There is never any "final word" or "definitive treatment" on this topic because new studies are always appearing, and adjustments must constantly be made to recommendations and advice that have gone before.

Because of the constant flux in this field, I find I must rely not only on my own reading and study, but also on the investigative skills of others if I hope even to approach the latest medical understanding of the topic. The main person who assists me in this research process is my professional literary collaborator, William Proctor. In addition, Bill has once again been instrumental in the organization and presentation of this book. As we have worked together on my books since 1980, Bill and I have learned a great deal from each other about how to handle stress in the world of writing and publishing books!

My primary business partner on the publishing scene—a man who has been the quarterback in honing book concepts and managing the business side of my book writing and other media projects—is my good friend, adviser, and literary agent,

Herbert M. Katz. Along with his colleague and wife, Nancy Katz, Herb has done a magnificent job of helping me spread the word of preventive medicine throughout the world.

For many years, my secretary and administrative assistant, Harriet Guthrie, has coordinated my book efforts, administrative work, busy travel schedule, and other responsibilities. There is no doubt that Harriet has made my professional life much easier and more relaxed. More than anyone else, she has helped me minimize the job stress that I confront daily. In fact, Harriet could have written her own version of Chapter 7, which deals with stress at work!

When it comes to minimizing negative stress in relationships, I must turn with thanks to my family—my wife, Millie, my daughter, Berkley, and my son, Tyler. They have provided an unparalleled "relaxed" support system of the type described in Chapter 8.

Finally, I continue to be grateful for the tremendous publishing operation at Thomas Nelson. The editors and other publishing specialists there have been extremely helpful in fine-tuning my manuscripts in the past, and I look forward to a continuing relationship with these fine professionals.

PART ONE

THE
GREAT PARADOX
OF STRESS

CHAPTER 1

WHAT IS THE PARADOX PRESCRIPTION —AND HOW CAN IT TRANSFORM THE STRESS IN YOUR LIFE?

Stress presents us with a profound paradox—a Jekyll and Hyde of health that can both heal and kill.

In its most menacing form—as wrenching emotion, physical trauma, or even chemical imbalance in the body—stress may pose a severe, if not deadly, threat to health. We all are familiar with the negative physical and mental fallout from fear, anger, deadline pressure, bodily injury, or allergic reaction. People who fail to adapt to such stresses may become ill or even die. In fact, many physicians and scientists—myself included—believe that bad stress, in one form or another, lies at the heart of many of our health problems.

But stress can also put on a friendlier face. For example, you have probably tasted the thrill of prevailing in a close sports contest or other game. Or you may have experienced the exhilarating drive and sense of expectancy arising from a string of successes at work or on a personal project. Or you may know the energizing edginess from a well-controlled rush of adrenaline, which produces your best performance in a speech or interview.

In its positive incarnations, stress provides a boundless source of inner power for achievement, happiness, and well-being. The challenge, however, is to minimize the ravages to health of negative stress and, at the same time, to release the healing, productive energy of positive stress.

Can Stress Heal? is my response to this challenge. Put simply, the basic healing principle in this book involves *not* trying to eliminate all bad stress because that just isn't possible. The threat to health lies not in the stress itself, but in the way you react to it. So your goal should be, paradoxically, to

- *accept* bad stress as inevitable, yet
- develop a resilience of mind and body that allows you to react positively to bad stress—and perhaps even turn it to your advantage.

In practical terms, how can you achieve this result? A recent harrowing experience I had on the South China Sea suggests the potential of the Paradox Prescription.

High Stress on the High Seas

With a Filipino guide on board, I plunged through the white-water rapids in a dugout canoe, deep in a tropical jungle a few hours' drive from Manila. We had some tense moments as the roiling river waters swallowed our bow, and I had to hold on for dear life to avoid being swept overboard. I still don't know how we avoided capsizing, but the experience was exhilarating, and I was left with a pleasantly drained sense of fulfillment.

As we were driving back to Manila, I felt I had probably reached my peak of good physical stress and excitement for the summer. After that diversion, I was ready for what I expected would be a calm, uneventful cruise on our luxury liner, which was waiting for us in the Manila harbor. I couldn't have been more wrong.

Every year, I lead a summer excursion to educate laypeople and medical professionals in the principles of preventive medicine. As part of the program, the participants also work on improving their personal fitness and diet programs. Our ship was fitted for every taste in exercise, including a selection of indoor equipment and an expansive seventh-deck walking-jogging track, with 3.7 laps to the mile.

This particular year, I was scheduled to deliver my lectures as we steamed from Manila to such exotic ports as Taipei, Naha in Okinawa, and Shanghai. Everything seemed under control and proceeding according to plan until just after the Philippines faded from sight over the horizon. At that point, the waves began to build, first ten feet, then fifteen, then higher and higher—and the gentle sea breeze turned into a steady forty-mile-per-hour gale.

The captain soon revealed the mystery behind the abrupt weather change. He announced that the cause of the turbulence was our ship's position about four hundred miles from the eye of Typhoon Zane, a monster storm that was moving steadily in a northeasterly direction over open water and packing winds up to 150 miles per hour.

The captain tried to assure us that we were well out of reach of any danger. But our twelve-deck cruise ship was already rolling and tossing violently, and increasing numbers of the nine hundred passengers and six hundred crew were getting queasy. Needless to say, no one was willing or permitted to risk walking or jogging on the severely pitching seventh deck. It was getting hard enough to stay on your feet in the staterooms.

My wife, Millie, and I had been assigned to one of the worst locations on board, with quarters on the eighth deck at the bow of the ship. Only a hull was between us and the pounding ocean. We could feel every wave crashing against the vessel. Not only that, the bow exaggerated all the ship's movements, up and down, back and forth.

Soon, Millie became quite ill, and I started getting nauseated, even though I usually don't suffer from seasickness. Illness can exacerbate the fears accompanying a storm at sea to the point that calm, reasonable human interactions become almost unbearable. So I braced for plenty of frustrations and complaints to emerge in our relationship, as well as in those with other passengers.

But despite her gastrointestinal distress, Millie responded like a real trooper, as did most of the other passengers I encountered. The prevailing concern seemed to be focused on what the storm might do, not on temporary physical discomfort.

Still, I knew that it was imperative to make sure all of us suffered as little as possible from the nausea. To counter the illness, the ship's staff recommended that we place acupressure bands on our wrists. The Chinese believe there is an acupressure point just below the crease on the wrist that, if pressed, will relieve an upset stomach. To my surprise, despite the initial skepticism I felt as a Western-trained doctor, the technique actually helped. Also, we began to take regular doses of the medication Antivert.

With my physical situation stabilized, and with Millie experiencing some degree of relief, I was able to turn to our tour group. Most were suffering from seasickness, and some needed medical attention. After passing out the extra acupressure bands, I administered various medications.

"This is turning into a hospital ship!" one of my seasick patients remarked. That comment was more prophetic than he realized.

After about twelve hours, we pulled into port in Taiwan, and I expected that our next stop would be China and the port of Shanghai, which would take us even farther from the path of Zane. But the captain said that we would lay over in Taiwan for only a few hours and then would have to head back out into the ocean in a northeasterly direction toward Okinawa—and the typhoon.

"Is that wise?" we asked.

"I would rather go to Shanghai first," he replied. "But for political reasons—namely, the problems between China and Taiwan—we can't go directly to Shanghai from here. We have to go to Okinawa first."

Also, he said, we needed to discharge some of our passengers in Okinawa and pick up some new ones in the port of Naha. I didn't like the plan when I first heard it, and I liked it even less when we were out on the open ocean again. Although the typhoon was moving in our direction at only 6 to 8 miles per hour, we were traveling toward it at a speed of about 22 miles per hour.

Within a couple of hours, the weather conditions deteriorated dramatically. We found ourselves only 220 miles from the eye of the typhoon, with winds on deck approaching hurricane speeds of 75 miles per hour. The waves, which were reaching heights of fifty-five feet, were literally exploding over the bow at the precise spot where Millie and I were supposed to be sleeping.

It was obvious we were courting disaster. The bow of the ship would rise to incredible heights. Then, like a giant seagoing roller coaster, the vessel would smash down into the water with such force that it felt and sounded as though it were being ripped apart. Elsewhere in the ship, windows were shattering, tables and chairs were slamming into walls, and at least one TV set shook free from its mounting and crashed to the floor.

"The captain has ordered all passengers to stay in their staterooms—and hang on to something solid!" a junior officer reported to us. Our cabin steward was too sick to relay the message.

Millie clung tightly to the bedpost. Quite frankly, I was worried about her condition as she grew progressively more nauseated. But I felt I also had a responsibility to check on our other passengers who might be in more danger. After securing the consent of the ship's officers, I moved about the decks, bracing myself against bulkheads and railings, and I was shocked at what I found.

The physical shambles created by the storm was bad enough, but the condition of the people was of far greater concern. Everywhere I looked, I saw bruises and lacerations. Three people had broken bones—one, a fractured arm; another, a cracked collarbone; and a third, a shattered wrist. Everyone, even the most seasoned sailors, seemed to be throwing up.

As I assessed the situation, I mulled over an argument that I would make to try to convince the captain to turn the ship around. Neither the passengers nor possibly the ship could stand much more punishment.

But before I could intervene, the captain made an announcement that afforded some relief. He said he had received permission to go to China directly, without first passing through Okinawa—a fortunate decision since Typhoon Zane was at that moment directly over the island. So we could change direction and hightail it away from the typhoon.

Unfortunately, the rest of his news wasn't so good. He told us we had to chug around in the open seas for another twenty-four hours because the Chinese would not agree to receive us until the next day. More politics! We had already fought the elements for nearly thirty hours.

It didn't help that one of the passengers was a former navy man who had been spreading stories about how he had faced typhoon-level winds during a Pacific voyage in World War II.

"We lost 750 people in that storm," he said. It was clear that he was quite concerned that the same thing might happen to us.

A general sense of alarm and stress was building among the passengers. I did what I could to comfort and reassure them. But like the high winds and waves that were beating against us, the anxiety didn't really subside until we reached Shanghai and the mouth of the Chang River some twenty-four hours later.

I certainly wasn't immune to the anxious atmosphere. For one thing, I was worried about the health of my wife, who was extremely nauseated. I was also deeply concerned about the welfare of the passengers in my tour group, who had embarked on the trip with full confidence in my leadership. As for my safety, I was constantly aware of the threat to life and limb. But an unusual physical and emotional calm had come over me—and at first, I couldn't figure out why.

The Calm During the Storm

In the past, I had encountered stressful situations on ship voyages, such as a perilous North Sea storm off the coast of Norway. The winds were so violent, I feared we would crash into nearby drilling rigs and punch a hole in our hull.

Even worse, on another occasion my family and I were crossing one of the gulfs of Tahiti in a fragile ferryboat during a pitch-black night when a storm kicked up and nearly caused us to capsize. Someone suggested we might sing to calm our nerves, and I thought the most appropriate song might be "Nearer, My God, to Thee"!

I don't hesitate to admit that in those situations, I was really scared. Furthermore, the fear for myself and my family triggered some rather serious changes inside my body—primarily because I am what is known as a "vascular reactor."

Confessions of a Vascular Reactor

Physical and emotional challenges such as the threat of Typhoon Zane can pose peculiar physical and emotional challenges to a person with my health profile. One reason is that I am a classic type A personality: task-oriented, ambitious, workaholic, perfectionistic, fast-talking, and impatient. After Dr. Meyer Friedman, who heads his own stress institute at Mount Zion Medical Center in San Francisco, identified this category, I immediately saw that I fit the description to a T.

You know people like me. They easily become exasperated when confronted with colleagues who disappoint, with delays that upset carefully laid itineraries, or with unexpected events that require adjustments of crammed daily schedules. Usually without a minute to spare, they devote large chunks of life to managing heavy professional pressures and fulfilling numerous responsibilities.

Such personalities feed on pressure, personal challenge, and a full schedule. They always need a full plate of activity, or they get restless or bored. Often, the self-induced pressure and activity involve *positive* stress in the sense that the stress moves the person toward success and adventure—and tends to produce genuine enjoyment and joie de vivre.

But dangers lurk in the background for type A personalities. For one thing, positive stress may turn sour if there is too much of it. If I pack my schedule too full, or if I allow my approach to my daily agenda to become too rigid, I can expect to feel stressed out. That involves a conscious sense of being anxious and out of control, and unhealthful physical changes may accompany the feelings, including a temporary rise in blood pressure.

Too many times, I allowed my schedule to become so crowded that my health literally hung in the balance. The reason involves a second factor in my health profile: I am what is known as a "vascular reactor."

In brief, this condition involves an abrupt spike or upsurge of blood pressure, usually when the person experiences some type of stress. The rise may affect the upper (systolic) number of a blood pressure reading, the lower (diastolic) number, or both numbers.

As a result of this tendency, when I become tense or over-loaded—or even when I anticipate a stressful situation—my blood pressure increases. For example, even though I have given hundreds of speeches, sometimes to audiences numbering in the thousands, tension still builds inside my body before a public appearance. Frankly, it's somewhat annoying that I continue to get stage fright at this point in my life. You would think that a professional lecturer would be as comfortable on the platform as in his living room!

On the positive side, of course, some stage fright, with accompanying changes in your cardiovascular response, is a benefit in helping you to perform better. But too much tension, including even temporary high hikes in blood pressure, can be bad for your health.

Such vascular reactivity can appear during all sorts of stress. For example, some people with this condition are sometimes said to have "white coat hypertension" because of their tendency to experience a spike in pressure when a doctor (wearing a white coat!) is about to conduct an exam.

I have seen my blood pressure go up on a portable monitoring device before I gave a speech or participated in another high-stress event. Fortunately, twenty-four-hour monitoring devices have shown that my blood pressure readings are usually within the normal range. In other words, medically speaking, I am not currently suffering from the disease of hypertension.

This condition is fairly common, but vascular reactors ignore blood pressure volatility at their peril. Among other things, there is evidence that a person whose pressure tends to shoot upward too often is at a slightly higher risk of developing permanent hypertension than someone with more stable blood pressure. Permanent hypertension can lead to stroke and other serious health problems. So it's extremely important for people like me to take countermeasures to manage stress and reduce cardiovascular risks.

On the chemical level, excessive stress triggers the release of various fight-or-flight hormones, such as epinephrine (adrenaline) or norepinephrine (noradrenaline). In addition to helping raise blood pressure, stress hormones can cause the heart to beat abnormally fast, induce irregular heartbeats, and possibly produce excess free radicals. These extra unstable oxygen molecules have been linked to cancer, heart disease, cataracts, and scores of other illnesses.

I found myself facing a challenge on several fronts, emotional as well as physiologic, as the winds of Typhoon Zane beat against our vessel. But fortunately, the vascular reactor was prepared.

The Vascular Reactor Meets Typhoon Zane

The winds and waves on the South China Sea were stronger than those I had encountered in the North Sea or in Tahiti, and on the current voyage I was witnessing considerably more illness and injury. But my emotional and physiologic responses were quite different.

First, I felt relatively calm inside. To be sure, I was deeply concerned about the physical threat as the waves exploded over the decks and the winds howled and battered us. Also, I felt a responsibility to do my best to combat injuries and illnesses. And as the leader of our tour, I did all I could to influence the captain to get out of the path of the storm. But believe it or not, I was never conscious of being afraid or nervous about the outcome.

Second, I know that my heart never raced during the entire experience. Rather, it continued beating within normal ranges, even when I was tending to passengers or fighting to keep my balance on deck.

Third, I know my blood pressure didn't rise precipitously, as it often had during stressful moments in the past.

Why the positive changes in my mind and body?

In retrospect, I realize that many of the powerful stress-management principles that had become established in my life were operating in full force to keep me calm and in control of myself. These factors are essential components of my Paradox Prescription Program, which we'll be discussing in detail in Part II of this book. In brief, here are some of the specific "prescriptions" that were working for me on board that cruise ship.

Nature's Best Tranquilizer—Aerobic Exercise

One reason that my heart rate stayed steady and my blood pressure failed to spike upward was the cumulative effect of aerobic, or endurance, exercise. I became known as the "father of aerobics" after the publication of my first book, *Aerobics*, in 1968, and I've always tried to practice what I preach. For more than thirty-six years, since experiencing a fitness conversion around the age of thirty, I have engaged in running, jogging, fast walking, or some other aerobic activity at least four days a week, typically for at least thirty to forty minutes per day.

The physiologic effect of such activity on a vascular reactor like me is well documented in medical literature. Typically, if a fit person exercises aerobically an hour before the measurement of blood pressure, the systolic (upper number) reading will be lower during the exam. In other words, the tendency of the vascular reactor's blood pressure to spike as a result of the white coat phenomenon is minimized.

In a related finding, the 1988 Consensus Conference on Exercise, Fitness, and Health summed up the long-term benefits of endurance exercise on high blood pressure this way: "Individuals with essential hypertension can decrease their resting systolic and diastolic blood pressure by approximately 10 mm Hg with endurance exercise training."

(For more on this prescription, see Chapter 4.)

The Mystery of Molecular Balance

Outside pressures and actions may produce multiple stresses on the molecular level in the body. The more we can reach a healthy balance with these forces, the lower the risk of various diseases will be.

As I have already mentioned, the particular molecular threat I was facing on the cruise experience was the release of excess free radicals, unstable oxygen molecules that may be produced by emotional and physical stress. Paradoxically, we need free radicals for efficient bodily functioning, but too many can contribute to many serious diseases, including lowered immune function. My physical fitness, in addition to certain spiritual and psychological coping mechanisms (see more on this later), minimized my internal physiologic stress and my risk for developing disease.

(Refer to Chapter 5 for more detail on this principle.)

The Mind-Spirit Solution

As I always do in a crisis situation, I sought divine help when the storm first hit us. I prayed we would all get through it alive and in safety. But the answers to my prayers did not come quite as I had expected (that has happened with many of my significant spiritual experiences).

For example, when I prayed the first time, I really believed that God would keep us safe. But when I heard the captain's announcement about another twenty-four-hour delay and possibly more storm exposure, I began to wonder what God was doing. When I realized that we would have to go through more battering after what we had already endured, I was almost tempted to pray, "Let me die and be done with it!" The ordeal we were facing was that bad.

My feelings of discouragement were fleeting, however, and my conviction that God would pull us through was strong. So the prayer I offered went something like this: "Lord, I don't want to go through this for another twenty-four hours, but if we have to, help us handle it. Let us get to port without any more injuries or problems."

The winds and waves didn't calm down until we reached Shanghai and the mouth of the Chang River. But with those spiritual resources, we were given the strength and hope to pass through the second crisis. Also, in what I saw as a direct answer to all of our prayers, the incidence of sickness, injuries, and fears subsided.

(See Chapter 6 for more on how to make use of these mind-spirit support systems.)

The Principles of Release and Retreat

In the simplest terms, this aspect of the Paradox Prescription, which can be applied to many other areas of life, including work and personal projects, involves psychological coping mechanisms.

As you can see from my description of the crisis, I consciously released any belief that I could control the situation. Much of our unhealthy response to stress arises from *trying to control what is beyond our control.*

At the same time, I evaluated my position in relation to that of the captain and asserted myself as much as I could in my dealings with the crew. The medical literature on this subject makes it clear that strategic assertiveness—which involves taking the initiative without embracing anger—is an important tool for controlling stress.

My suggestions about the route we should have taken may or may not have had any impact. But from the viewpoint of lowering my stress, it was extremely important for me, in a calm and reasonable way, to speak my mind to those who had control over decisions that would affect my life and the lives of those in my care.

(For more applications of these and other practical devices for coping with stress, see Chapter 7.)

Relaxing in Relationships

When you are thrust into a position of serious responsibility with family members and others depending on you—and the situation carries potentially dangerous consequences—remaining calm is difficult. Yet I have found that, paradoxically, the more pressure I am under in such circumstances, the more I need to relax in my relationships. Much, if not most, of the stress in our lives—as well as the health problems that result—comes from a failure to manage stressful relationships successfully. (You'll learn more about reducing stress in difficult relationships in Chapter 8.)

Making it through a difficult passage in relationships may require the application of numerous coping devices, including one approach I call the Paradox of Worst Expectations. It involves expecting and preparing for the worst from those around you in a crisis—yet knowing that you are likely to be surprised by a brand of courage and inner strength in others that may well surpass your own.

As the threat of Typhoon Zane increased, I consciously began to expect the worst of those around me: I imagined the most unpleasant responses that were possible with my patients, my colleagues, and my wife in the crisis, and I prepared mentally to withstand them.

They surprised me in many cases by responding with patience, hope, and even optimism in the face of the storm's threat. In fact, as the Paradox of Worst Expectations suggests, they often showed more strength and equanimity than I felt I possessed.

Other facets of the Paradox Prescription, including medically based stress-reduction techniques and practical exercises, will be detailed in later chapters. But here is a sampling of the additional topics to which you will be introduced:

- The Longevity Paradox—which is based on the idea that to live long and well, with a maximum of inner peace, you must live for each moment.
- The Faith Paradox—a particular spiritual response to stress that involves a package of paradoxical principles. These include modern medical applications of such time-honored truths as "The least will be greatest," "The leader

will be servant," and "You must lose your life in order to save it."

- The Paradox of Release and Retreat—which is part of my scientific response to the physiologic stress produced by pressures at work. Many of us have soaring dreams and ambitions about what we would like to accomplish in this life. Yet practical experience—as well as findings in the research literature—establishes beyond any doubt that to achieve and succeed, we must constantly back off. We must release our goals in order to reach them, and we must retreat from important work in order to become fully productive.

- The Doctor-Patient Paradox—a stress-management principle that urges you to be under the regular care of a physician but, at the same time, to take the initiative and collaborate with your doctor.

You are almost ready to begin to design your own Paradox Prescription Program. But before we embark on an exploration of how you can apply the Paradox Prescription in your life, you need to understand more about the distinction between positive and negative stress, including ways that the bad may be converted into the good.

CHAPTER 2

MOVING FROM NEGATIVE TO POSITIVE STRESS

This book is designed to provide you with personal access to the Cooper Paradox Prescription Program, an action-oriented set of strategies that will enable you to *immunize* yourself against the harmful effects of stress.

In this chapter, you will learn about the harm that may arise from bad stress. So brace yourself. What you are about to read will, for the most part, present a rather grim picture of various ways that stress can threaten your health and life. But I'm a great believer in the principle that you must know your enemy before you can fight effectively. And make no mistake: Stress *is* your deadly enemy, which you must learn to combat with all the resources at your disposal.

The first step in understanding bad stress is to grasp the basic meaning of stress itself: What exactly is it, and how do the experts define it?

A Brief Definition of Stress

In scientific terms, *stress*—both good and bad—has been defined by the late stress researcher and guru Hans Selye as the body's "nonspecific response to any demand made upon it." That is, when you are exposed to a stressor—or an influence that causes stress—you can't expect your body to react with a clear, identifiable pain or discomfort. Rather, there will tend to be a more general or indirect reaction, which typically involves the shifting of some chemical balance deep within your system.

Suppose, for instance, that you encounter negative stress, such as problems in your marriage or another close relationship. When bad stress hits, the body does *not* react as it might to a blow or other physical injury, with pain, bleeding, or some other limited and directly related result. Instead, your system responds in a more general way, such as through the release of hormones, including adrenaline, cortisone, and related secretions produced by the adrenal glands near the kidneys.

These chemical changes, in turn, may cause more forceful pumping of blood from the heart, a higher heart rate, and a rise in blood pressure. After a series of such stress reactions over a period of months or years, your body may "adapt" to produce permanent hypertension, heart disease, or other diseases.

Clearly, assuming that these responses are unimportant just because they are nonspecific would be unwise. A generalized, nonspecific reaction may be more powerful than the blood and pain accompanying a wound.

To evaluate the balance between good and bad stress in my life, a fairly simple rule of thumb that I follow is this: If the demands in my daily routine are keeping my interest in life honed to a sharp edge, infusing me with a sense of excitement, and not eroding my energy levels, I assume I am experiencing *good* stress. But if the pressures are causing me to feel tired, distracted, anxious, confused, or upset, I know I am involved with *bad* stress. At that point the alarms begin to go off in my head.

Now, to alert you to how stress may flash danger signals for your health, here are some of the most important symptoms of negative stress that I've encountered in my more than four decades of medical practice.

What Are the Main Symptoms of Negative Stress?

A reported two-thirds of Americans have said that they feel stressed out at least once a week, according to a national survey released in 1995 by *Prevention* magazine. But what are the signs of bad stress that appear in the bodies and minds of such people?

To help you identify the presence of negative stress, I've listed several telltale symptoms that may appear in your body and mind. This is certainly not an exhaustive list. But whenever I notice one of these common stress signals in a patient, I know that person is probably wrestling with stress-related health risks.

Stress Symptom #1: Fatigue

Late in 1994, Harvard University President Neil Rudenstine was overcome by fatigue and pressure from his demanding duties and had to take off three months to rest. Reportedly a micromanager, Rudenstine had focused on the minutiae of his massive responsibilities of administration, fund-raising, and alumni hand-holding. He wrote seemingly countless notes to students and faculty members. He attended endless parties, meetings, and other functions. And finally, he ran out of steam.

As President Rudenstine's fatigue grew, he overslept, and he dozed off in meetings. To cope with his fatigue, he had to take a leave of absence and seek medical help. When he returned to his duties at the beginning of March 1995, *Harvard Magazine* editorialized in these terms:

> Happily, President Rudenstine's medical problems appear to be contained. But . . . the issue goes beyond questions of personality—how much energy Rudenstine's hands-on style consumes and whether he can adjust his own throttle. Instead, it concerns the challenges of governing Harvard. (March-April 1995, p. 27)

Stress Symptom #2: Back Problems

The most accurate description of what happened to Duke University basketball coach Mike Krzyzewski is that he hit the wall—emotionally speaking. The highly successful forty-eight-year-old Krzyzewski had led the Blue Devils to two NCAA national championships, as well as several finalist and Final Four appearances. Then, he had to undergo back surgery in October 1994 for a ruptured disk—an injury linked to the stresses and strains associated with his job.

Krzyzewski said that even though he was able to overcome fatigue in the past, he became exhausted, sleepless, and fearful about the future condition of his health. As a result, he withdrew from his coaching post for the rest of the season. "It shows me that you can have limits, no matter who you think you are," he told *The New York Times* (March 7, 1995, p. 14).

Stress Symptom #3: Frequent Headaches

San Francisco Giants baseball stalwart Barry Bonds indicated at the end of the 1995 season that he was considering walking away from a contract that would earn him $8 million the following season. His reasons: He was under too much stress and had become sick and tired of being blamed for everything that was wrong with his team. Symptoms included migraine headaches in the morning and anger at the fans.

Stress Symptom #4: Weight Fluctuations and Gastrointestinal Problems

Shannon Faulkner, the first woman cadet to enter the Citadel military college in South Carolina, sued the college for admission and won. But during the more than two years of her successful legal fight, she said she gained fifty pounds and succumbed to the stresses and strains of the struggle. After spending time in a local hospital and undergoing tests for stomach pains, she gave up in September of 1995 and withdrew as a student.

These, then, are a few representative symptoms of negative stress. You can probably add your own special variations to this list, such as twitching muscles, generalized anxiety, or depression. Once you have isolated the typical ways your body and mind signal the presence of stress, you are ready to take the next step: You should find the *causes* of your bad stress. Then, when you understand the causes, you will be in a strong position to *fight* the causes and overcome the stress.

What Are the Causes of Negative Stress?

Almost anything can cause bad stress because, as you already know, bad stress is determined largely by how we react as individuals to outside pressures and concerns. For example, a given work assignment may involve positive stress for one person because the challenge motivates and exhilarates. But the same assignment may trigger negative stress for another individual who feels overloaded or threatened by the responsibility.

Bad stress can arise from almost any quarter, even from seemingly minor or insignificant events or worries. Nevertheless, several significant stress-triggers, or stressors, in life can initiate bad stress in almost everyone. I classify them as major and minor because of their relative ability to produce intense, bad stress in most people. But as you'll see, some of the so-called minor stressors can wreak havoc with the bodies and emotions of those who lack strong stress-coping mechanisms. If you encounter any of these stressors, major or minor, you can assume that a negative stress reaction won't be far behind.

The Major Stressors

The following three categories of stress-triggers have been shown time and time again to have the ability to raise stress levels significantly in most people.

Major Stressor #1: A Great Personal Crisis

According to the Holmes Life Change Score—based on a classic questionnaire devised by Thomas H. Holmes, an American psychiatrist—the five most stressful events you can experience in life include the following:

- The death of a spouse
- Divorce
- Marital separation

- Detention in a jail or other penal institution
- Death of a close family member

Many of my patients suffering from depression, anxiety, and other emotional problems have recently gone through one of these crises.

Major Stressor #2: General Job Stress

The highest-profile, highest-pressure jobs, such as those held by Harvard's Neil Rudenstine and Duke's Mike Krzyzewski, present obvious difficulties with negative stress. But practically every job has the potential to generate stresses and strains that cause emotional and physical problems. Juliet Schor, the Harvard researcher who authored *The Overworked American,* has concluded from her most recent research that job stress is the number one pressure afflicting adult Americans. This complaint ranks higher than the traditionally cited stress of financial worries. (see *The Wall Street Journal,* October 20, 1995, p. B1.)

Furthermore, high pay is no respecter of pressure. The legal and medical professions, which pay some of the highest salaries in the United States, have been associated with particularly high levels of stress.

The New York State Bar Association has become so concerned about the problem that the organization recently published a thirty-page booklet entitled *Handbook on Stress Management for Lawyers* by Dr. Ellen I. Carni, a clinical psychologist. Among other things, Dr. Carni cites a 1990 survey by the American Bar Association that shows the number of lawyers who were "very satisfied" with their jobs dropped 20 percent in six years. The latest figures show that barely one-third of attorneys are very satisfied in their profession.

The reasons that lawyers give for their mounting stress and lack of happiness include longer working hours, less time with their families, tremendous pressure to be promoted to partner, and the low esteem in which the public holds their profession.

Physicians are also prone to high levels of stress—with the result that medical mistakes may multiply. Many times, the errors have a strong connection to work overload, fatigue, excessive pressure to perform well, and a lack of sleep.

A case in point: A Connecticut doctor was roused from his home in the early morning hours to perform delicate brain surgery to remove a clot. An hour into the operation, he discovered that he had been working on the left side of the man's skull, but the clot was on the right side! The patient survived, but an investigation was immediately launched and was continuing at the time of this writing.

Major Stressor #3: Difficult Age-Related Transitions

Some of the most serious health concerns arise as we move from one major age transition to another. For many of my patients, illnesses and other health complaints seem to escalate as a woman goes through menopause, a man faces declining sexual potency, or an older worker deals with forced retirement. In most of these transitions, stress seems to play a major role in posing a threat to health.

The teenage years are perhaps the most difficult transition time in life. Dramatic changes in the body and the emotions occur against a backdrop of raging hormones and uncertainties about the future and the meaning of life.

With such pressures it's understandable that suicide has become a major cause of death among American teenagers, along with auto accidents and homicides. Furthermore, the problem seems to be getting worse: According to the Centers for Disease Control and Prevention, the incidence of suicides among teenagers and young adults nearly tripled between 1952 and 1992.

These tragic statistics become quite personal when they involve someone like Scott Croteau, a high school football star and A student from Maine. Scott was being courted by Ivy League recruiters, and in general, he seemed to have everything going for him. But then, in September of 1995, he was found hanging by his neck from a cherry tree, with a .22 caliber bullet hole in his right temple.

The state medical examiner determined that Scott killed himself in what amounted to a double suicide. In other words, he used two methods to be sure that he was successful.

Why did Scott take his own life? An in-depth investigation by *The New York Times* revealed one common thread, which emerged from interviews with those who knew Scott well: It was evident that he felt under tremendous pressure to perform to perfection. Apparently, in the midst of the excessive, self-generated stress syndrome, something snapped inside, and he decided he just couldn't live with the pressure any longer.

The stresses of advancing age and serious illness can lead to depression and to related emotional and physical problems, such as suicide and stroke. A 1994 report of the New York Task Force on Life and the Law determined that doctors generally do a poor job of alleviating suffering and depression among dying and chronically ill patients. Only about half of all the cancer patients studied received adequate pain or depression treatment. As a result, there was a relatively high incidence of suicidal feelings among those patients. But when they were given proper treatment—and the physical and mental stresses on them were reduced—they usually abandoned their wish to commit suicide.

These three major stressors—involving great personal crises, serious job pressures, and difficult age transitions—are almost certain to produce physical or emotional symptoms in persons who lack the ability to cope properly with stress. But two other secondary, or minor, stressors can also create problems.

The Minor Stressors

The following two sources of stress—jury duty and regular exposure to urban traffic—tend to be somewhat less serious for most people than the major stressors we have just considered. But under some circumstances, these seemingly minor influences can produce significant negative physical and emotional responses, and for a few people they may prove to be just as powerful as the major stressors.

Minor Stressor #1: Jury Duty

Huge segments of the population have served on juries and in the process have found themselves exposed to excessive stress. The results can affect blood pressure, heart rate, and other physical functions. That's why I always try to ascertain exactly what life experiences my patients have been going through just before they come in to see me for an exam.

Although the circuslike atmosphere surrounding the O. J. Simpson double-murder trial is perhaps the most obvious example of how jurors can be placed under unusual stress, ordinary trials can also exert tremendous pressure.

Many studies have found that jurors exposed to evidence of violence, intense publicity, or racial tension during a trial will display classic signs of stress, such as depression, anxiety, weight loss, sleep loss, a tendency to cry frequently, and problems with personal relationships. Thomas Hafemeister, an attorney and psychologist with the National Center for State Courts in Williamsburg, Virginia, has conducted one such study and has concluded that stress on jurors is not only a source of personal irritation and suffering, but is also a potential threat to the very foundations of the jury system.

In a similar vein, a 1993 survey of 312 jurors in Dallas revealed that people who served as jurors in high-stress trials were six times as likely as nonjurors to experience the symptoms of depression (from a *Los Angeles Times* study reported in *The Miami Herald,* September 24, 1995, p. 14A).

Minor Stressor #2: Exposure to Traffic

Some of my angriest patients are those who are exposed on a regular basis to the frustration, noise, and pollution associated with urban traffic. If you are a commuter, you should always take that into account when you are evaluating your health and learn better ways to lower your stress reactions to heavy traffic.

Stress related to traffic has increased along with the nationwide increase in population and vehicles. Between 1960 and 1990, there was a 39 percent growth in the national population, and during the same period, the number of vehicles per household increased from 1.03 to 1.67. Simultaneously, complaints about traffic-related anxiety and other emotional problems have soared.

Traffic stress has been the subject of regular, formal study since the late 1970s, when Raymond W. Novaco, a psychologist and professor at the University of California at Irvine, began his intensive research. Among other things, Novaco has found that traffic pressures can raise blood pressure, lower a person's tolerance for frustration, and interfere with job stability.

Also, in a 1992 study he conducted on the link between traffic and aggression, Novaco concluded that freeway shootings tended to be triggered by the *cumulative* effects of traffic stress over several weeks or months. More than 40 percent of male drivers and up to 21 percent of females he interviewed acknowledged chasing an offensive driver.

Miami clinical psychologist Eric Goldstein also noticed a decided upturn in traffic complaints beginning in the early 1990s. Today, he finds that traffic stress is one of the two or three most common complaints among his clients. (see *The Miami Herald,* October 16, 1995, p. 1A.)

• • • •

To understand what goes on inside the human body when pressure builds up from any stressor, consider the experience of a businessman whom I will call Clark.

Clark's Complaint

Clark had been working with his company for nearly ten years, and he was reaping executive benefits. He enjoyed a six-figure salary, a lucrative pension and profit-sharing arrangement, good medical benefits, and a large expense account.

But Clark was not happy—not by a long shot. His main complaint was that his new boss had made it clear that all personnel and systems in the corporation were to be reevaluated. Nobody's job or method of operation was secure. The reason for the pressure, according to the CEO, was that profits had not been high enough, and productivity had been lagging.

To add to his stress, Clark had personally been called on the carpet at a recent meeting of top executives because his division was performing below the chief executive's expectations. As he listened to the criticisms of his work and that of his team, Clark said, his stomach "began to churn" and his blood "began to boil." He could also feel his heart racing throughout the encounter.

At the beginning and end of the meeting, Clark sensed that he wanted to literally run away. He would have done anything to have avoided going to the meeting in the first place, and after it was over, he wanted to "disappear." But in the middle of the meeting, as the attacks were being leveled against him, his feelings were different. He became more angry and aggressive, and it was all he could do to hold his tongue and keep from lashing out at his boss.

The best way Clark could describe his emotions was that they moved in a cycle. First, he felt high anxiety; then, anger took over; and finally, his emotions returned to an even deeper fear and sense of uncertainty about his future.

What exactly was going on in Clark's body as the feelings surged inside?

On a superficial level, his feelings were mirrored in his face. As he walked into the conference room and his anxiety soared, his face took on a drawn, pale look. His heart beat faster, perspiration formed on his forehead, and his breathing became rapid and shallow.

Soon after the meeting started and his anger rose with the mounting criticism, Clark became angry, and his cheeks and neck became flushed. Then, after the confrontation was finished and the CEO's harsh spotlight shifted to someone else, fear and worry about his future took over.

By the time he walked out of the meeting, Clark was emotionally and physically drained, drenched with sweat, and even more pale and drawn than when he entered the room. Thoroughly washed out by the time he arrived at home that night, Clark started running a fever. He had to stay home the next day because of the onset of flulike symptoms.

A physiologic volcano

Clark's intense feelings had roots well below the surface signs and symptoms. His outward manifestations were only the tip of a physiologic volcano smoldering deep inside his body.

The biochemical explanation of his responses can be summarized like this: The intense pressures and circumstances—or stressors—that he faced triggered the release of certain "stress hormones." These chemical secretions included adrenaline (epinephrine) and noradrenaline (norepinephrine), which are produced by the adrenals, the endocrine glands located next to the kidneys.

The operation of these two hormones differs in ways that may explain some of Clark's outward responses during his meeting. Typically, adrenaline floods the body when a person is fearful or anxious, with the result that certain blood-channeling capillaries are shut down: hence, the paleness of Clark's face as blood was squeezed away from the skin. In contrast, the levels of noradrenaline increase dramatically when a person becomes angry, and the chemical reactions can cause the face and neck to become flushed.

Despite these differences, for the most part adrenaline and noradrenaline tend to behave similarly in the body. Among other things, they constrict blood vessels, cause the heart to pump faster, and produce other changes known as the fight-or-flight response. Such chemical changes were originally designed to prepare the body to handle straightforward challenges, such as responding to a weapon-wielding human enemy or fending off attacks of wild beasts.

In earlier times, such confrontations could be resolved rather quickly, either by running away or by standing one's ground and fighting. When the stressor—the enemy or animal—had been left behind or vanquished, the "revved up" body would return quickly to normal.

Our more complicated culture makes dealing with enemies and pressures a more subtle affair. Consequently, more time and effort are needed to resolve our kind of stress than what was demanded by the stress faced by our ancient hunter-gatherer ancestors.

In a situation like the one confronting Clark, it just isn't possible to dispose immediately of the pressures connected with the unpleasant boss or work environment. Instead, such stress can hang on for days, weeks, months, or years. Furthermore, as we have seen earlier, the persistent stresses and strains may cause the body to adapt, or change permanently, often in extremely unhealthy ways. The end result may be life-threatening disorders, such as high blood pressure, heart disease, or a weakened immune system.

Where Clark's Stress— or Yours—May Be Heading

What are the potential difficulties that Clark and the rest of us may face if we fail to take steps to counter bad stress? The following overview will introduce you to a few possibilities.

Decreased Natural Immunity

In addition to the excessive production of adrenaline and noradrenaline, the stress that Clark was feeling probably triggered the release of a hormone known as CRH, or corticotropin-releasing hormone. CRH is a peptide hormone that originates in the part of the brain known as the hypothalamus. According to researchers at the National Institute of Mental Health, reporting in the British medical journal *Lancet* (July 1995), this substance may stick to cells and set off a series of chemical changes that result in an altered gene. The changed gene, designated as a "POMC gene," is thought to have the power to help viruses and cancer cells grow stronger and multiply. Such an ominous mechanism may have accounted for Clark's lowered immunity and increased susceptibility to flus and viruses.

Stress can also lower immunity in other ways, such as through sleep disturbances. Typically, a person under heavy stress will have trouble getting a good night's sleep. A study on sleep at the Department of Psychiatry, University of California, San Diego, showed that the activity of natural "killer" (immune) cells dropped by 28 percent in healthy but sleep-deprived male participants.

The twenty-three volunteers, who were tested over a three-day period, were allowed to sleep eight hours the first day, but they were kept awake between 3:00 A.M. and 7:00 A.M. the second day. After the second sleep-deprived night, the killer cell count declined significantly in eighteen of the participants. On the third day, after a final night of good sleep, the killer cell activity returned to normal.

The researchers, who published their findings in the November-December 1994 issue of *Psychosomatic Medicine,* concluded that even short-term loss of sleep may severely affect the body's immune function. A further point of interest: This sort of sleep disturbance is a typical characteristic of depressed patients, who experience lower than average levels of immunity.

Heart Attacks

The scientific evidence has established clearly that out-of-control stress in a person like Clark is linked to a higher risk of heart attacks. For example, in the November 1994 issue of the American Heart Association's journal *Circulation,* Dr. Ichiro Kawachi of the Harvard School of Public Health reported that men who complain of high anxiety are four to six times more likely to die from sudden heart failure than men who are less anxious.

Dr. Kawachi said that excessive psychological stress may cause "electrical storms" in the heart, which can lead to fatal irregular heartbeats. He based his findings on data compiled at the ongoing Veterans Affairs Department's Normative Aging Study, which began in 1961 and has included 2,280 men in the Boston area.

In a related study, reported in the October 1995 issue of *Circulation,* other Harvard doctors found that the risk of a heart attack doubled in the two hours following an episode of anger. The study, which included both men and women, determined that the most frequent causes of this heart-threatening anger were arguments with family members, conflicts at work, and legal problems.

What occurs in the body during such anger? The scientists noted that anger increases the flow of adrenaline, which, as we have already seen, increases the heart rate and blood pressure. This hormonal surge in the body can cause fat-based deposits of plaque to break off from blood vessel walls and form blood clots. As a result, vessels leading to the heart may become blocked.

Increased Blood Pressure

Clark's stressful job situation may also contribute to permanent hypertension. Researchers at the Cardiovascular and Hypertension Center, New York Hospital-Cornell University Medical College, reported in October 1994 that employees who reported experiencing significant job strain had systolic blood pressure that was on average nearly seven points higher than employees who felt under less pressure.

Stomach Pains

Clark may not have stomach problems yet, but the pressures in his life definitely put him at risk. A 1994 study at Vanderbilt University School of Medicine, which focused on 197 children with chronic abdominal pain, revealed that those who faced stressful situations at home and school had more stomach problems than the young people with more positive life experiences. The stressors exerting negative influences on the children included an inability to fit in socially with their peers, and parents who were burdened by various physical problems.

Asthma

Asthma is another potential threat to highly stressed people like Clark. There may be an emerging epidemic of asthma in one of the most pressured living environments in the nation, the South Bronx in New York City, according to a study published by *The New York Times* on September 5, 1995. The National Institutes of Health have reported that between 1983 and 1993, there was a 34 percent increase in the prevalence of asthma. Furthermore, the South Bronx has been identified as one of the nation's most seriously afflicted urban areas.

The exact reason for the epidemic? Several experts, including New York epidemiologist Dr. Kevin Weiss, point to family stress that is aggravated in overcrowded urban settings. The Bronx, in particular, has New York City's highest proportion of households with more than one person per room. Specifically,

16.6 percent of all Bronx households are in this category, in contrast to 12.3 percent in New York City as a whole.

Premature Births

All of the health dangers cited here can afflict women as well as men. But pregnant women under pressure at work face an additional threat. Stresses and strains on the job—including high levels of noise, long periods of standing, and work-weeks of more than forty hours—significantly increase the risk that pregnant women will give birth to premature babies, according to a study of more than 1,400 nurses by the University of Michigan. The report, which appeared in the September 15, 1995, issue of the *American Journal of Obstetrics and Gynecology*, revealed that nurses under heavy stress were 70 to 80 percent more likely than other women to deliver premature, underweight babies.

One reason that my attention has been riveted by such medical conditions is that I see stressed-out patients every day. *Most* of the illnesses I treat at the Cooper Clinic in Dallas—including heart problems, high blood pressure, immune system deficiencies, and cancer—seem to have a stress component.

So now, having run the gamut in our consideration of bad stress and its effects, how can we take steps to transform that bad stress into good stress? The answer begins in Chapter 3.

PART TWO

THE COOPER PARADOX PRESCRIPTION PROGRAM

How to Write Your Own Paradox Prescription

It's time for you to learn how to write your own Paradox Prescription against stress.

In the previous chapter, you were introduced to the general types and effects of bad stress. Now, we'll get more personal. How do you go about identifying your own particular stress problems, and what practical steps can you take to overcome them?

What Are Your Main Stressors?

My program for immunizing you against bad stress begins with an identification of your main stressors. As you know, stressors are the primary influences, both external and internal, that make you feel stressed out, with such symptoms as fatigue, anxiety, depression, a sense of being at loose ends, or various physical aches and pains.

I recommend six questions to help my patients identify their major stressors. Ask them of yourself to ascertain your current stress status.

Question 1: What causes me to experience intense negative emotions, such as worry, irritability, anger, depression, or a sense of being overwhelmed by life?

This question underlies all the others. If you can answer it precisely, your search for your greatest sources of stress will become much easier.

Use this approach: Go over your daily schedule, hour by hour, for seven consecutive days. As you proceed, note on a piece of paper each influence that seems to produce the most significant negative emotional responses. Focus especially on disturbing feelings that linger for more than a few minutes.

For example, suppose you discover that your business meetings with one particular client or colleague "set you off" more than discussions with other people. You may feel angry or distracted for a half hour, an hour, or even longer after one of these sessions. By pinpointing such a significant source of stress, you have taken the first important step toward solving the problem. Now, you can take countermeasures, such as avoiding the individual entirely, or employing one of the "depressurizing" tactics described in Chapters 6, 7, and 8.

After completing this evaluation of a typical week in your life, you will be in a better position to highlight your most serious causes of bad stress as you move through the remaining questions.

Question 2: What situations or pressures tend to cause me to experience physical problems, such as fatigue, an upset stomach, headache, backache, or muscle tension?

As we saw in the previous chapter, a stressful situation or influence may produce certain symptoms in your body or emotions. If you experience these symptoms soon after encountering one of the potential stressors you listed in answering Question 1, that's a good sign that you have uncovered a serious stress-producing factor in your life.

Question 3: Does something seem to trigger disturbances in my sleep patterns? If so, what is the offending factor?

Occasionally, you may be unable to go to sleep easily, or perhaps you wake frequently during the night. Or maybe you wake too early in the morning and are unable to get back to sleep because your mind is racing, going over the impending day's schedule.

First, see if you can identify a possible stress-related source for such sleep disturbances. Then, try to eliminate other potential nonstress causes, such as prostate trouble, which may cause men to make frequent trips to the bathroom during the night. If you find that a nonphysical stressor is the likely culprit for your sleep problems, check Step #2 later in this chapter for ways to overcome it.

Question 4: What causes me to become preoccupied or distracted when I am trying to concentrate on an important task or attempting to spend quality time with a family member, friend, or business colleague?

Usually, a preoccupation or distraction that gets in the way of personal tasks or important relationships is a first sign of stress. It may also be the first step toward anxiety, depression, and other medical problems. So be alert to any difficulty in your ability to concentrate or focus.

Question 5: What excuses do I give when I miss an exercise session?

During the more than four decades that I have been practicing preventive medicine, I have probably heard more excuses for not exercising—or for interrupting an exercise routine—than anyone on earth:

- "My office load is too heavy right now."
- "I have to attend to some pressing family matters."
- "I'm committed to doing volunteer work that takes up all my free time."
- "I can't exercise after work because I don't leave the office until dinnertime."
- "I can't get up early because I'm working so late."
- "I am just too tired these days to exercise."

Such comments usually signal a routine that is at high risk for stress-related problems—whether the particular stressor is related to work, volunteer commitments, or family. Furthermore, this temptation to avoid or skip personal fitness sessions poses one of the major paradoxes in this book:

Exercise is usually the first thing we neglect when we are under stress. But regular exercise—including aerobic (endurance) activity, stretching routines, and strength work—

is exactly what the busy, pressured person should *always* include in his or her packed daily schedule. (For more, see Chapter 4.) In short, the multiple health-enhancing and stress-reducing benefits of physical activity are too important to neglect.

Question 6: What tempts me to skip my daily devotions or spiritual meditations?

Like physical exercise, spiritual exercise is one of the most powerful antidotes to stress. Yet pursuing a regular spiritual discipline often presents us with another paradox:

Spiritual stability is a must for a stress-free life. But when certain pressures become intense, one of the first things most people eliminate is their daily devotions, meditations, or other times of creative solitude.

In 1535, the Reformation leader Martin Luther wrote to a man named Peter Beskendorf—or "Peter the Barber" as he was called—because Beskendorf asked Luther for advice about how to pray. Luther explained that when he didn't feel at all like praying—or when he thought he was too busy to pray—such feelings were powerful signals that he should spend extra time in prayer. In those circumstances, Luther reached for his psalter and rushed to the privacy of his room or the sanctity of the church where he would meditate on the Ten Commandments and other Bible verses.

Clearly, Luther understood that when the pressures of his daily life grew burdensome, it was imperative to rely even more heavily on his spiritual resources. Or as he put it in Reformation terms to Peter the Barber, "the flesh and the devil always prevent and hinder prayer."

Let me pass on a piece of advice that I've learned both in wrestling with my own stress problems and in advising my patients: It's always best to *write down* your responses to these six questions and then put the list in an accessible spot for safekeeping. This way, you will always have at hand a comprehensive overview of the main stressors in your life. Also, the specific itemization will be invaluable as you begin to write your personal Paradox Prescription for stress.

Although I have to go over these six diagnostic questions periodically, I have reached the point in my life where I know by heart my main sources of stress. In a word, almost all of my pressure problems can be traced to aspects of my work.

My Personal Search for Stress "Immunization"

My daily schedule is a constant juggling act, with at least five full-time careers vying for my attention.

First, I'm a professional lecturer with scores of speaking engagements around the world every year. Most people I know who make their living as speakers give no more presentations than I do—yet this is only one of my careers.

Second, I'm chairman of the board of trustees and chief fund-raiser for the Cooper Institute for Aerobics Research. This role requires me to keep in regular touch with potential donors and attend many board and committee meetings.

Third, I'm chief executive officer of the Cooper Clinic and Aerobics Center in Dallas. This sprawling set of facilities on almost thirty acres, with more than three hundred employees and an annual budget of close to $20 million, has provided health and recreational services for tens of thousands of people from all over the world.

Fourth, I'm a practicing physician with a full patient caseload. This involves not only giving exams, prescriptions, and advice to individuals, but also dictating patient reports and monitoring charts every day I'm in the office. Like most other physicians, I respond to emergencies for my regular patients, and whenever possible, I'm available to advise them on the phone.

Fifth, I author a new book every eighteen months to two years. This book you are now reading is my fifteenth, and there is no end in sight. If anything—with medical challenges and questions escalating on all fronts—the demand seems to be increasing for more, rather than fewer, popular publications on preventive medicine.

To top it all off, I constantly strive to adjust my work schedule so that I can make sufficient time available for my family, friends, and church activities. Just trying to find leisure time is an ongoing source of stress for me!

I cite this litany of commitments not to boast, but to confess. Taking on too much is probably my greatest weakness— and my greatest source of negative stress.

Yet paradoxically, the very work that can on occasion stress me out is also one of my most significant sources of satisfaction. I tend to take on too much not because I'm a masochist, driven to inflict pain on my body and psyche, but because I really love what I do. Deep down, I guess I'm afraid I'll miss something enjoyable and fulfilling if I try to lighten my workload.

My primary challenge has been first to ask the right questions so that I can identify precisely my most serious sources of stress. Then, I have proceeded to design a personalized program that enables me to fight my worst stressors, and that means achieving a more balanced approach to work.

In practical terms, my personal fight against stress—which I also call my "stress immunization"—involves seven steps. These constitute the basics of the Paradox Prescription Program that I recommend to my patients and to you as well. In brief, here they are:

Step #1: Assume a paradoxical mind-set.

Step #2: Build a foundation of healthy sleep.

Step #3: Take regular doses of "nature's best tranquilizer"—aerobic and other physical exercise.

Step #4: Learn to fight stress on the molecular level.

Step #5: Erect a powerful mind-spirit defense perimeter.

Step #6: Become an expert in using "depressurizing tactics" in daily high-stress situations.

Step #7: Get regular medical stress checkups.

I'll go into some detail in this chapter about the first two steps of the Paradox Prescription, which focus on the paradoxical mind-set and laying a foundation of adequate sleep. Subsequent chapters will explore the remaining five steps.

Step #1:
Assume a Paradoxical Mind-Set

To succeed in minimizing and controlling the bad stress in your life, you need to prepare your mind and body, almost as a soldier would for battle. In effect, you must get ready for a fight—but a special kind of fight.

So far, in describing my basic approach to bad stress, I have used some rather assertive and even confrontational terms, such as *fight, combat,* and *immunize.* But rather than try to smash your opponent head-on, as you might in football or boxing, with stress you would do well to think more in terms of the ancient Japanese fighting art of *jujitsu,* a word that comes from a Chinese root meaning "soft" or "gentle."

Although jujitsu was transformed earlier in the twentieth century into the more aggressive sport of judo, the philosophy behind the older fighting style is more suited to the way you should deal with stress. As the name implies, *jujitsu* was known as the "gentle art" because it was based on the principle not of trying to meet force with force, but of turning an opponent's force and strength against him.

In other words, if a person pushes, you give way instead of pushing back; you might even pull him faster in your direction. But then, using an adept defensive move, you use his momentum to trip or throw him to the mat.

My approach to handling stress is a form of mental jujitsu. I believe in pursuing the fight systematically and forcefully, but not with a full frontal assault. Instead, I usually battle through less direct, flanking maneuvers.

To put this another way, you may sometimes have to learn to outwit your stress by employing unexpected weapons and techniques, including certain approaches that are best expressed in terms of a paradox. This indirect kind of fighting is the essence of what I call the "paradoxical mind-set." Here are some illustrations that you will encounter later in this book:

- An emotional paradox: By embracing stress—through understanding it and accepting it as an integral part of life—you can often cause it to disappear.
- A fitness paradox: When you are feeling stressed out, you should upset your body's balance by pushing yourself physically so that you become temporarily uncomfortable. This discomfort will, in turn, lead to long-lasting improvements in your health and energy.
- A creativity paradox: If you stop pushing a tired, over-loaded mind to create, you will trigger greater creativity.
- A success paradox: If you let go of your ambitions, you will achieve the ambitions more easily with much less pressure.
- A productivity paradox: Retreating from work will enable you to become more productive. In a way, working less may produce better results!
- A relationship paradox: Good relationships that have the lowest levels of stress are rooted not in complete peace and tranquillity, but in controlled conflict.
- A spiritual paradox: True spiritual serenity and inner strength emerge when life seems most unsettled.

One reason I prefer such a paradoxical mind-set as I face daily challenges is that a more aggressive, confrontational style usually backfires. Fuming at or wrestling with a stressor is quite likely to make things worse.

For example, suppose you allow yourself to become increasingly angry and tense with a supervisor at work who is putting pressure on you to meet an impossible deadline. As his unreasonable demands intensify, you become angrier still, and you end up exploding and hurting your case as well as your emotional balance. You may begin to suffer more serious signs of stress, such as rising blood pressure or other physical problems.

Certainly, it's natural to meet aggression with aggression, anger with anger, and fire with fire. But suppose you choose a less predictable approach by responding to this annoying supervisor quietly and calmly. For example, you may refrain from lashing out to protect yourself. Also, you could ask your boss to sit down with you to discuss the possibility of restructuring your deadline or his work expectations.

If both of you can find a mutually acceptable solution, so that the required work can be finished in a more reasonable time frame, you will have found a strong weapon to combat your stress. Incidentally, you will also have learned the power of an ancient biblical paradox: "A soft answer turns away wrath."

It's essential to start your stress response program by resolving to change the way you initially think and react to stressors. Always avoid responding without thinking. Cultivate the habit of taking a deep breath. Discipline yourself to put your first idea on hold and to look for fresh ways to solve the problem. Jot them down when they pop into your mind. Then sleep on the matter for at least one night.

When you return to your consideration of that stressor after a good night's sleep, you may find that your first idea or your natural response was the right one. But more likely, you'll discover that the best solution is unexpected and may even involve a paradox.

The essence of the paradoxical mind-set, then, is to avoid trying to shoot from the hip at the stress in your life. But this is just the beginning of the Paradox Prescription. The next step in building a solid wall of protection against stress is healing your body and mind through quality sleep.

Step #2:
Build a Solid Foundation of Sleep

When I encounter a patient who seems tired or under significant stress, one of the first things I ask is, "How well are you sleeping?"

Like good nutrition, good sleep is a topic often overlooked by the average physician, usually because we doctors aren't given much training on either subject in medical school. When a person comes in with a complaint, we automatically tend to evaluate physical or emotional symptoms, diagnose the probable condition or illness, and then prescribe some technological treatment, such as medication, surgery, or other standard procedure.

Yet poor sleep may not just be part of the problem that causes or exacerbates stress; it may be the *whole* problem. I'm again reminded of that surgeon who was called at home in the early morning hours to perform brain surgery and started to operate on the left side when he should have been operating on the right side.

Fortunately, the patient recovered without ill effects, but what caused the doctor to make such a mistake?

Several possible factors were cited, including the fact that the patient had a bruise on the left side of his face, which caused the doctor to think the brain injury was just above that point and, as a result, to operate on that side. But apparently, the CAT scan results, which the doctor had studied, were clear. For some reason, he overlooked them. (See the Associated Press report, published in *The Miami Herald,* September 14, 1995, p. 10A.)

Why did this near tragic mistake occur? The only explanation that seems to make sense is that the doctor had been roused from his home and called upon to operate during hours when most people would have been asleep. Most likely, he was unusually tired and at the same time was being forced to operate outside his "circadian rhythm," or the natural twenty-four-hour sleep-wake cycle to which his body was accustomed. A lack of sleep will inevitably aggravate the stress that always accompanies a difficult job assignment, such as doing brain surgery.

But the interaction between stressful events and sleep may vary from one person to the next. A 1995 study at the Stanford University School of Medicine compared the levels of stress of forty-two good sleepers and forty-two bad sleepers. The median age of the participants was about sixty-eight years.

Their responses to the stressors were quite different. Those with higher life stress had greater difficulty falling asleep than did those with lower life stress. (See *Psychology of Aging*, September 1995, pp. 352–7.)

One possible conclusion from these results is that the sleep patterns of some people are more sensitive to stressful influences than are the patterns of other people. Also, the study suggests that a chronically poor sleeper tends to be less successful in coping with stress than a good sleeper, even when the stressors of the two people are similar.

In other words, different people may react in completely different ways to the same types of stimuli. Or as I have already suggested several times in these pages, "good" and "bad" stress—including the symptoms of "bad" stress, such as insomnia—are determined more by how we respond to our stressors than by the stressors themselves.

So if you are a poor sleeper or if stressful influences tend to have a particularly negative effect on your sleep patterns, what are some of the health implications?

Medical studies have shown that sleep deprivation and the stress related to it can have numerous devastating effects on the human body, for example:

• A decline in the immune function

You will recall that the 1994 study at the Department of Psychiatry, University of California, San Diego—which we discussed in connection with Clark in the previous chapter—revealed that sleep disturbances are associated with a reduction of natural "killer" cell activity, which is related to human immunity.

Such research suggests that the human immune function is directly linked to sleep problems, some of which may result from excessive bad stress. Fortunately, there is no mystery about a powerful antidote that can readily restore full immunity: Just reduce your stress and get more sleep!

- A decline in mental performance and hormone production

Most people sense that they don't think or perform as well when they have slept poorly. Scientific support for these feelings can be found in a 1994 study of prolonged physical stress, sleep deprivation, and energy deficiency in young Norwegian military cadets.

The researchers from the Norwegian Defence Research Establishment, Kjeller, Norway, evaluated the circadian rhythm of hormones and mental performance of twenty-eight cadets throughout a five-day military training course. During the exercise, they engaged in heavy physical activity corresponding to 35 percent of their maximum ability to process oxygen, and they had almost no food and sleep.

As a result of the regimen, the cadets experienced severe decreases in hormones, including testosterone, thyroid-stimulating hormone, and DHEA (dihydroepiandrosterone). Also, mental performance decreased. After four to five days of rest, most functions returned to normal. (See *European Journal of Endocrinology,* July 1994, pp. 56–66.)

• A disruption of the adrenal systems

Stress seems to have a kind of domino effect on the body's fight-or-flight hormones, which are produced by the adrenal glands. An important piece of health that "topples" when the adrenals get out of whack is the ability to sleep.

Researchers at the University of Texas Medical Branch, Galveston, reported in 1995 that either physical or psychological stressors can increase the production of the corticotropin-releasing hormone (CRH), which is produced through the adrenal system. CRH, in turn, operates to keep a person awake. (See *Advances in Neuroimmunology,* 5 [1995], pp. 127–43.)

Any type of insomnia can wreak havoc with our health, but some types are more dangerous than others. In general, medical experts have identified two main categories of sleeping problems: chronic and reactive. Chronic insomnia, which is the most serious, will receive our attention first; then, we'll move on to the more common reactive type.

The Challenge of Chronic Insomnia

The chronic problems include long-term sleep difficulties arising from serious or established medical conditions, such as these:

• Sleep apnea

As you age, the chances increase that you may suffer from this breathing disorder, which may affect more than one-third of people over age sixty-five. This problem arises from a collapse of the tissues at the base of the throat. Although this condition usually just causes interruption of sleep, it can be fatal in the most severe cases. Symptoms may include shallow breathing, difficulty in breathing, and very loud snoring.

If you think you have this condition, see your doctor for treatment. In mild cases, sleeping with your head raised may be enough. In more serious situations, he or she may prescribe throat surgery or the insertion of a device to facilitate breathing.

• Congestive heart failure

This condition involves leakage of fluid into tissues, such as the lungs and legs, because of inadequate pumping of the heart. Shortness of breath, excessive fatigue, swelling of the legs, or restless sleep may be symptoms, especially if the fluid is collecting in the lungs.

Obviously, your physician must treat this problem. Possible responses include ACE inhibitors (e.g., Vasotec®), which are normally used for hypertension, and diuretics, which reduce the levels of fluid in the body.

• Urinary problems

Older men may find their sleep interrupted because of an enlarged prostate, which makes it necessary to urinate more frequently during the night. Women may experience a descended uterus or other changes in the reproductive system, which can promote more trips to the bathroom.

But even if you don't have one of these problems, you may wake up more often than you would like because you are drinking relatively large quantities of liquids before bedtime. The solution: Try cutting your consumption of drinks in half and see if that helps you sleep better through the night.

- Restless legs syndrome (RLS) and a related problem known as "periodic limb movement disorder"

An estimated 10 percent of people over age sixty-five and 5 percent of all adults have restless legs syndrome, which involves constant or uncontrolled movement of the legs while sitting, lying in bed, or sleeping. Possible medical solutions include such drugs as the benzodiazepines, L-dopa, or codeine.

- Ongoing emotional problems, such as clinical depression

Depression, anxiety, or other emotional disturbances that cannot be linked to a particular stressor or source of pressure may create sleep problems but should be treated with medications or other therapy by a qualified physician.

• Natural aging

As we grow older, our patterns of sleep change. In general, older people tend to go to bed earlier, get up earlier, and sleep for shorter periods at night. On the other hand, they often need naps during the day to enable them to get their full complement of sleep.

These changes are nothing to worry about. The best response is to "go with the flow" of your life: Plan on getting less sleep at night, and then plug a nap in sometime during the day. I usually sleep only five to six hours a night. But then occasionally, I'll take a brief nap on the sofa in my office in the middle of the afternoon. By conforming to my changing sleeping patterns in this way, I get all the shut-eye I need without fighting the natural shifts occurring in my sleeping rhythms.

The stress-reduction responses described in this chapter may relieve these chronic sleep problems to some extent. But if you have any of the symptoms mentioned in this discussion, you should definitely consult with your physician, who will likely prescribe special medications or other treatments. One new possibility is known as "LEET therapy."

LEET therapy

Patients with chronic insomnia may benefit from a treatment known as low energy emission therapy (LEET), according to researchers from Symtonic USA, Inc., in New York City. (See *Sleep*, May 1996, pp. 327–36.)

In this study, 106 patients with chronic insomnia were treated twenty minutes during the late afternoons, three times a week, for a total of twelve treatments, with electromagnetic fields conducted through a mouthpiece or with an inert mouthpiece. The group that received the active treatment experienced a significant increase in total sleep time.

The researchers concluded that LEET is safe and tolerated well by patients and can effectively improve the sleep of chronic insomniacs, who are handled like those in the study. If other methods suggested in this section for improving your sleep don't work, you might ask your doctor to check into LEET, which could be effective for some people because the electrical currents may affect brain waves or neurotransmitters (brain chemicals). Or you might look to the Far East for even more exotic solutions to your problem, such as acupuncture.

Acupuncture

Scientists at the Department of Physiology, Shanghai Second Medical University, China, have found that acupuncture is a simple and useful treatment for insomnia, with a success rate of approximately 90 percent. (See *Science and Clinical Neuroscience,* May 1995, pp. 119–20.)

The acupuncture points vary according to the practitioner, but the usual points used are known technically as "Shenmen" (HT7) and "Anmien" (extrapoint).

Caution: Before you try acupuncture, be sure that you are dealing with an experienced practitioner who has a solid track record of therapeutic successes and also medical references approved by your physician.

Such formal treatments may not be necessary for you, especially if you suffer only occasional sleep difficulties.

How About Treatments for Reactive Insomnia?

In contrast to the chronic conditions we have been discussing, reactive sleep problems are characterized by short-term sleeplessness, which, as the name implies, results from *reactions* to a wide variety of circumstances, or stressors. These may include sleeping in an uncomfortable bed; having jet lag; and experiencing various personal, family, or job-related worries that may cause anxiety, depression, or other emotional upsets.

Reactive insomnia, which typically lasts for a limited period of time—ranging from one night to as long as two to three weeks—can often be treated through short-term, practical stress-reduction techniques. Here are some of the possibilities that have been established in the scientific literature or in clinical practice:

Music

Some people doze off more easily when soft music is playing in the background. But music just *before* bedtime may prove to be even more important.

In a study published in the *Journal of Holistic Nursing* (September 1995, pp. 248–54), researchers studied twenty-five elderly participants who had complained of sleep disturbances. The patients were directed to listen to music, including classical pieces, just before bedtime, and they kept daily logs to evaluate the effectiveness of the musical approach. The results: Twenty-four out of the twenty-five participants, or 96 percent, reported improved sleep after this music therapy.

Hot baths

Researchers at the Sleep Disorders Center at the McLean Hospital, Belmont, Massachusetts, conducted a 1996 study to evaluate passive body heating—mainly from hot baths—for treatment of insomnia in older adults. At the outset of their report, Dr. C. M. Dorsey and several colleagues noted that an increase in body temperature in adults early in the evening through such means as hot baths has been shown to produce an increase in slow-wave sleep in the early part of the sleep period. This condition promotes sounder sleep.

In Dorsey's study, which involved a two-night testing period, nine female insomniacs, aged sixty to seventy-two years, were given hot baths 1.5 hours before bed on the first night. Then, they received lukewarm baths 1.5 hours before bed on the second night. The hot baths measured 40.0 to 40.5 degrees Celsius (about 104 degrees Fahrenheit), and the lukewarm baths, 37.5 to 38.5 degrees Celsius (about 100 degrees Fahrenheit).

The researchers found that the hot baths improved sleep continuity and encouraged an increase in slow-wave sleep patterns. The participants reported that they experienced significantly "deeper" and more restful sleep after the hot baths. In addition, the hot baths delayed the lowering of body temperature during the night for the participants.

Aerobic exercise

The experiences of thousands of patients I've treated at the Cooper Clinic over the years have impressed on me the value of aerobic or endurance exercise as a means of overcoming insomnia. This kind of exercise includes such repetitive-motion activities as walking, jogging, cycling, swimming, cross-country skiing, and even low-impact aerobics and brisk walking.

You should follow several guidelines to maximize the sleep-enhancing effects of this method:

- Do not perform any vigorous, sweat-producing exercise within two to three hours of bedtime because such activity may keep you awake.
- Exercise regularly—at least three to four times a week, and a minimum of twenty minutes per session. If you work out less frequently, the sleep effects will be minimized.
- Avoid engaging in competitive events if you are trying to improve your sleep. Many older competitive athletes I've known tend to "replay" races or other sports events in their minds, especially on the day of the competition. That heightened mental activity can overcome the beneficial physical effects of the exercise.
- Finish off your workout with a hot bath or shower. Remember the previous point that hot baths just before bedtime enhance sleep.

Why does aerobic exercise done in this fashion work so well as a sleep-inducer? Although the mechanism is unclear, some researchers have suggested that the release of endorphins, which are morphinelike neurotransmitters produced in the brain, may help relax the body and tranquilize the mind. Whatever the reason, there is no doubt that regular aerobic exercise has proven to be a powerful "sleeping pill" for many people.

Nutritional therapies

Several reports assert that increasing the intake of the amino acid tryptophan just before retiring can help overcome insomnia. Tryptophan, which has been designated as an essential amino acid because the body can't produce it, helps trigger the release in the brain of the neurotransmitter serotonin. Serotonin, in turn, governs human moods and behavior and has been associated with the relief of insomnia and stress.

You can get extra tryptophan in your food through milk, red meats, seeds (especially sesame and sunflower seeds), poultry, cottage cheese, and canned tuna in water. Over-the-counter tryptophan supplements were banned by the Food and Drug Administration (FDA) a number of years ago after a contaminated supply got into the market.

My nutritional therapy suggestion for insomnia would be this: Try having a cup of skim milk and perhaps a small turkey, tuna, or chicken sandwich just before you go to bed. This should be enough to trigger the release of extra tryptophan and serotonin in your system.

Other possible nutritional responses to insomnia include taking supplements of magnesium, pyridoxine (vitamin B^6), and thiamine (vitamin B_1). Some research has suggested that small doses of melatonin may help with insomnia. But before you try any of these remedies, check with your physician. (For more on this subject see my *Advanced Nutritional Therapies*

[Thomas Nelson, 1997], especially the entries in Part II for "Amino Acids," "Insomnia," and "Melatonin.")

Prayer and meditation

Experts in relaxation therapy, such as Dr. Herbert Benson of the Harvard Medical School, have reported great benefits from prayer and meditation just before bedtime. The most effective approach seems to involve repetitive and meditative prayers, such as turning a short passage of Scripture over and over in your mind. Or, as the psalmists suggested, you might meditate on God's "promises," "laws," and "wonders." (See especially Ps. 119.) The idea is not to do hard, analytical thinking about religion or philosophy at night. Rather, you should hold the principle or verse in your mind. Also, as you consider the passage or promise, allow random thoughts to drift in and out of your consciousness, without trying to confront them directly. (Remember the jujitsu analogy.)

According to Benson, this method helps to block out the worries and concerns of the day, produces a physiologically identifiable "relaxation response" (with such effects as slower heart rate and lower blood pressure), and paves the way for peaceful sleep. (For more, see Benson's *Beyond the Relaxation Response* [Berkley, 1985], pp. 133–6.)

Elimination of stressors

This treatment is one of the most obvious but is often overlooked. If your sleep problems can be traced to a particular source or set of "loose ends" in your life, the best response may be to tie up the loose ends. I always recommend that before they do anything else, my patients should go over their stressor lists and then do everything in their power to eliminate or minimize their impact.

I find that my sleep is likely to suffer if I have an important decision hanging over my head. So my main objective will be to make that decision as soon as possible. When the decision is out of the way, I can expect productive sleep to return.

After years of suffering from interrupted sleep, I finally realized that a major factor keeping me awake at night was the fear that I would forget a certain idea or thought that popped into my mind. I have come up with a little trick to help me manage these nagging thoughts better: I now keep a blank pad of paper and a pencil next to my bed. Then, when I wake up at 4:00 A.M.—as type A personalities are likely to do on occasion—I can write down my thought and return peacefully to sleep with the assurance that I won't forget the pearl of wisdom. (Ironically, though, when I check what I've recorded the next morning, I find that, more often than not, the thought is useless or even ridiculous!)

Summing Up the Sleep Issue

To sum up, then, when you feel under stress, an evaluation of your current sleep patterns should be one of the first things you check. Poor sleep may be the sole cause of stress-related symptoms, like fatigue, anxiety, and depression. Also, a lack of sleep can cause other stressors to become blown totally out of proportion.

In this regard, I'm reminded of Carol, a full-time office manager and mother, who had become quite agitated by her husband's failure to take out the garbage and do other household chores on time. She would explode regularly and burst into tears when she found he was only a few minutes late in fulfilling these obligations—a reaction that seemed disproportionate to the offense.

Yet Carol's body confirmed that the stress in her life was taking its toll: Her last medical checkup had shown that her blood pressure had increased over the previous exam. During her checkup, she complained to her doctor that she was under too much pressure at home and at work, and that she wasn't getting enough help. As a result, she felt she had reached the breaking point.

There was no doubt that her domestic and career stressors were contributing to her problems. But her description of her situation somehow didn't seem to warrant her physical and emotional deterioration.

"Something else has to be going on with her," her physician said to a colleague.

Sure enough, a little probing revealed that Carol was sleeping poorly because of a "hidden" stressor. It seems that her newest child, a six-month-old with colic, was waking up several times a night, and the mother was the parent who always responded. As a result, her sleep was constantly being interrupted. She was only getting a little more than three hours of sleep a night, or less than half of what she needed.

Except for the new baby, everything else in Carol's life was essentially the same: She had always operated rather well as a full-time career person, mother, and wife. So it was clear that the arrival of the difficult new baby, and the resulting sleep deficiency, was the key factor that had made her other sources of stress unbearable.

The doctor communicated two possible solutions to the husband: First, he would have to take care of the baby for a few nights and let his wife catch up on her sleep. Then, the two of them could work out some sort of "baby-sharing" arrangement. Or they would have to hire a sitter at night, either permanently or until they could arrive at another acceptable solution.

Carol's husband tried handling the baby for a couple of nights, but he started becoming sleep-deprived. They settled on an arrangement where they alternated nights with the child. But once a week, they hired a sitter to watch over the baby so that both parents could rest. Fortunately, within another six weeks, the baby started sleeping through the night, and the parents were able to go back on a normal schedule.

This case illustrates a two-pronged way of dealing with sleep deprivation, which often works:

First, you have to identify a lack of good sleep as the culprit in your stress. Because sleep problems often hide behind other stressors, this initial step may take thought and analysis.

Second, the antidote to poor sleep may involve one or more of the medically established responses to sleep deprivation, such as hot baths or even doctor-supervised treatments and medications. Or you may just have to come up with an individual, practical solution that fits your particular situation, as Carol and her husband did.

In any event, when you know you are dealing with a stress problem, always look first at the possibility that sleep deprivation may be the underlying issue. If you begin to get more sleep, you may very well find that all your other stress symptoms disappear.

So Where Do You Stand in Writing Your Prescription?

Let's sum up where you are right now in writing your Paradox Prescription for personal stress immunization.

First, you know the basic questions to ask in order to identify the major stressors in your life, and you have spent time pondering them.

Don't skip over this procedure. You must be sure that you ask yourself these questions and come up with definite, realistic answers. Again, writing down your responses and keeping your stressors list in an easily accessed location will help you as you devise your Paradox Prescription strategy.

Second, you are now aware of the seven steps necessary to put together your Paradox Prescription Program, and you've considered in some detail the first two of these steps. Specifically, you know how to begin to protect yourself from negative stress by assuming a paradoxical mind-set and by building a foundation based on better sleep.

Now let's move on to Chapter 4, which deals with the next step in writing your personal Paradox Prescription—regular aerobic exercise.

CHAPTER 4

WHAT IS NATURE'S BEST TRANQUILIZER?

My day at the Cooper Clinic had been particularly stressful. I had just returned from a speaking engagement in the Northeast, only to be confronted with two media interviews, exams for a half-dozen patients, and several staff meetings. Physically, I was exhausted. Not only that, my back and legs felt achy; my thinking was fuzzy; and I was growing noticeably irritable and short with my colleagues.

The pressures of that particular day—and my symptoms in response to those pressures—pointed to one problem: a losing bout with bad stress. I was tempted to go home, have a good meal, and lie down in front of the TV set. But I knew that wasn't the right treatment for my problem.

Instead, I turned to the best natural tranquilizer I knew for bad stress at the end of a hard day of work—a physical workout, featuring a session of aerobic exercise. That meant running about two miles on the outdoor one-mile walking-jogging track at the Cooper Aerobics Center, which winds around trees and ponds just outside my office.

After changing into my exercise gear, I focused on the first part of my routine—a series of basic stretches. These included a lower-back routine, which involved lying flat on my back and pulling one leg up by the knee against my chest and holding a bent-knee position for about fifteen seconds. Next, I did the same movement with the other knee, and I pulled both knees up against the chest for a fifteen-second hold. In addition, I did hamstring stretches and other flexibility movements. (For examples, see my *Antioxidant Revolution* [Thomas Nelson, 1994], pp. 101–6.)

By the time I had finished about ten minutes of the stretches, I could already feel the pressures of the day dissipating. Yet I knew from experience that was only the beginning of my "natural tranquilizer" treatment. The next and most important phase was my aerobic or endurance workout, which involved jogging.

For the first half mile, I moved along rather slowly, probably at no more than a ten-minute-per-mile pace. Then, I increased to my normal cruising speed of about nine minutes per mile. (If I'm doing aerobic walking, which is part of my routine at least a couple of times a week, my speed is more like twelve minutes per mile.) For the first seven or eight minutes, I felt uncomfortable, almost as though I were pushing a wheelbarrow up a hill. As I continued, however, the running got easier until I almost sensed I was gliding or coasting.

As I neared the end of the session, I decided to push myself to go a little faster than usual. Slowly, I accelerated until I was running at a little less than an eight-minute-per-mile pace. For a short while, the increased speed made me feel exhilarated and supercharged. But then, the enjoyment faded. My breathing became more labored, and my body began to feel the strain. Rather than ratchet up the discomfort, I decided to decelerate to a slower comfort zone.

After I had finished my two miles, I walked for five to seven minutes as part of my "cool down" phase. I returned to the Aerobics Center gym and did a few strength exercises on the equipment we provide for our members. (Again, for examples, see my *Antioxidant Revolution,* pp. 106–16.)

The end result was that I was literally a different man after the workout. I was totally relaxed; my energy level had returned; I was thinking quite clearly; and perhaps most important of all, I was finding it easy to be pleasant to people once again. I was actually looking forward to meeting new members of the Center and putting in more time on my work after dinner.

In short, the exercise completely eliminated my bad stress. Certainly, I still was facing a great deal of work and plenty of professional responsibilities, but my *response* to those circumstances was transformed. I was experiencing good or positive stress, which was working to my benefit by making me more motivated, productive, and satisfied with life.

An Antidote for Headaches

Regular aerobic exercise also provides me with an antidote for stress headaches, which I get once or twice a week. Typically, I'll complain over the phone to my wife that I'm suffering from one of these pains, but I always resist taking medications because I prefer not to take drugs unless it's absolutely necessary. Instead, I'll go out at the end of my workday for a two- to three-mile jog. The headache tends to grow a little worse at the beginning of the run, but by the end, it always disappears.

When I finally arrive at home, my wife will ask me, "How's your headache?"

And I'll say, "What headache?"

As I reflect on these experiences, I realize what a paradox exercise poses as an antidote for stress. There is no doubt that athletic activity, especially aerobic exercise, is nature's best tranquilizer. It's the treatment of choice for most stress problems after a tough day at the office. Yet my first reaction at the end of a hard day is *not* to exercise, but to run in the opposite direction. In other words, I know what's best for me, but I resist doing it!

Why this paradoxical response?

How Exercise Helps You Transform Bad Stress

The answer is fairly simple: Any exercise, regardless of your experience or fitness level, can make you uncomfortable physically for a short time. It almost always takes up to eight or ten minutes before your body's systems adjust to a more intense level of movement and energy expenditure. Practically every time I go out for a jog, for instance, I feel like stopping and doing something else. The first quarter to half mile is not quite torture, but close enough to make me want to quit.

But then my attitude changes as I become more accustomed to a rapid heart rate, stronger blood flow, higher consumption of glucose (sugar) by the muscles, and increased processing of oxygen by the cardiovascular system. These and other changes project my body to a more active, yet pleasurable, "homeostatic balance," or stable level of operation.

Other important adjustments occur around the ten-minute mark: For one thing, I begin to feel the soothing, tranquilizing effects of the endorphins, or morphinelike neurotransmitters produced by aerobic exercise.

Just as significant, the hormones secreted by the adrenal glands during a stressful day—especially adrenaline, noradrenaline, and the corticoids—are in effect burned up by the exercise. Remember, these adrenal hormones were originally intended to prepare the body for a fight-or-flight response. Although they may be released through stressful influences, our bodies have been designed to eliminate them through active physical channels. Unfortunately, there often isn't any opportunity to get rid of excess accumulations of these substances during the normal, sedentary course of activities in today's "civilized" world of business and polite society. So, as we have already seen in Chapter 2, our bodies may adapt in unhealthful ways to the pileup of bad chemicals from bad stress, such as through higher blood pressure, release of excess free radicals, and other assaults on our physical systems.

Aerobic exercise is our most potent modern-day antidote to these destructive accumulations of stress. While I am engaging in my endurance workout, especially after about eight to ten minutes of continuous activity, I feel the stresses of the day slipping away.

How do I know when I am moving at an optimum pace to rid myself of stress?

I don't need a speedometer to check myself! Instead, I use a "breathe and talk" test. Because I have been working out for a number of years and have reached a relatively high level of fitness, I have found that while moving at about nine minutes per mile, I can breathe and talk without undue effort. This test signals when I am in an appropriate balance to obtain adequate aerobic benefits and, at the same time, to reduce the effects of stress in my life.

In fact, this concept of homeostatic balance points us toward the true meaning of *aerobics,* a term that I introduced to the world of exercise with my first book, *Aerobics,* back in 1968. *Aerobic* means literally "living in air," but when applied to endurance exercise, the term goes farther. The *Encyclopae-*

dia Britannica, fifteenth edition—noting that "the concept of aerobics was pioneered by physician Kenneth H. Cooper and popularized in his books"—describes *aerobics* as a

> system of physical conditioning developed to increase the efficiency of the body's intake of oxygen. Typical aerobic exercises (e.g., walking, running, swimming, dancing, and cycling) stimulate heart and lung activity long enough to produce beneficial changes in the body. To be effective, aerobic training must include a minimum of three sessions per week. During each session, the exerciser's heart rate must be raised to his training level for at least 20 minutes. (Vol. 1, p. 120)

To put this another way, aerobic conditioning improves the ability of the cardiovascular system to strike a healthy balance in processing oxygen. As you become more fit, you are able to take in and process increasing amounts of oxygen at significantly higher levels of activity.

The Importance of Being Uncomfortable

But there is at least one important qualification to this principle of aerobic balance: Remember what I said about my practice of occasionally increasing my level of activity to a point where I can't take in as much oxygen as I need. In this situation, I become *anaerobic,* or temporarily deprived of oxygen. Sprinters, basketball players, and other athletes who rely on short, intense bursts of speed or energy expenditure experience this anaerobic state. The typical physical response to an anaerobic effort is short-term physical discomfort.

Why do I subject myself periodically to this discomfort?

Again, another fitness paradox is buried in here—one that is directly related to the use of exercise as an antidote for stress. You've probably heard the old aphorism "No pain, no gain." The real meaning of this principle, at least as far as fitness is concerned, is that if you want to improve your condition—or as in my case, if you want to retard the natural decline in aerobic and physical power as you grow older—it's necessary to push yourself occasionally beyond your normal comfort zone.

I know if I always work out at exactly the same level, my overall fitness will decline with the natural process of aging. Yet as my fitness declines, so will my ability to produce endorphins, burn up the adrenal hormones, and otherwise overcome the effects of stress in my life. But if I push myself once or twice a week to exercise above my usual comfort zone, my decline in fitness will slow significantly. I may even increase my aerobic power, at least for a time. The temporary "pain" I feel will be a small price to pay for the additional protection against the effects of stress.

These personal reflections are my way of introducing you to the part of the Paradox Prescription that says a major line of defense against the stress in your life should be exercise. This means engaging in regular stretching, strength work, and *especially* aerobic activity. But I certainly don't expect you to base your entire natural tranquilizer program on one man's experience. Let's consider in more detail the scientific case for exercise as a superior antidote to bad stress.

The Scientific Case for Nature's Best Tranquilizer

Medical research continues to pile up in support of the power of exercise to reduce stress and stress-related symptoms. Here are some of the most recent findings:

• Regular aerobic exercise is a superior method for coping with stress.

In a 1996 study, Australian researchers from the Department of Psychology, University of Wollongong, New South Wales, compared the effects on stress of ten-week programs of aerobic exercise and relaxation training.

Sixty unfit male college students with no previous training in stress management were divided into four groups. Each group was assigned to one of these approaches: (1) a moderate aerobic exercise program; (2) a progressive relaxation program; (3) no stress-management interventions; or (4) group discussions, but no exposure in the group to any unusual stressors.

The first three groups were challenged by an acute stress experience that involved losing to a competitor of the opposite sex on a task requiring physical motor skills. The participants in the three groups received unpleasant information about their performance as an additional stressor.

The results: The aerobic exercisers, in comparison with the other groups, responded to the acute stress with more positive emotions, lower heart rates during the "competition," reduced systolic blood pressure, and superior motor performance. The group trained in progressive relaxation techniques also experienced a marked reduction in systolic blood pressure, but members did not show improvements in motor performance or emotional mood.

The researchers concluded that aerobic exercise is a superior strategy for coping with acute stress. (See *Behavioral Medicine*, Winter 1996, pp. 186–96.)

• Aerobic exercise can help conditions that may be stress-related, such as fibromyalgia.

Fibromyalgia, or fibrositis, is characterized by chronic and generalized aches and pains of several parts of the body, usually for three or more months at a time. Other symptoms include stiffness, tenderness, poor sleep, and fatigue. The precise cause of fibromyalgia is unknown, but stress and age appear to be factors.

In a 1996 study at the University Hospital of Trondheim, Norway, researchers compared the effects on fibromyalgia of short- and long-term training in three areas: aerobic exercise, special stress-management techniques, and ordinary medical care. Sixty patients were divided into the three programs for a fourteen-week study. They were checked during a follow-up exam at the end of four years.

The researchers concluded that both the aerobic exercise and the stress-management training produced positive short-term effects—though overall, aerobic exercise was the most effective treatment. (An interesting side issue: Aerobic exercise came in first in this short-term evaluation even though the patients were most skeptical at the outset about the possible benefits of exercise!)

The results changed somewhat at the four-year follow-up in that there were no obvious differences in severity of symptoms among the groups. The researchers noted that the slippage in the beneficial effects of aerobic exercise seemed to be due to a considerable compliance problem: The patients in the exercise group just didn't stick to their programs! (See *Scandinavian Journal of Rheumatology,* 1996, vol. 25, pp. 77–86.)

• Mild exercise is a preferred treatment for most short-term back pain.

Acute back pain—defined as discomfort lasting no more than three months, or temporary *sciatica* (pain that moves down the leg)—afflicts 80 percent of Americans at some point in their lives. Furthermore, as you know from Chapter 2, short-term back pain is a common symptom of bad stress.

Ninety percent of these people recover in a month on their own. But even though most of these problems are self-limiting, is there any way a patient can hasten recovery?

A panel of back specialists and consumers, assembled by the Department of Health and Human Services in December 1994, reported that surgery appears to help only one person in one hundred. Also, surgery is generally not justified within the first three months of the pain.

Instead, the experts prescribed low-stress exercises, such as walking, swimming, or biking, during the first two weeks of acute back pain. After that time, they recommended adding conditioning exercises for the trunk muscles (such as "crunches," bent-leg sit-ups, and other stomach work). For additional pain control, the scientists suggested the use of acetaminophen and nonsteroidal anti-inflammatory drugs, such as ibuprofen, naproxen, and aspirin. (See *The Wall Street Journal*, December 9, 1994, p. B5.)

• Aerobic exercise can help adults with mild to moderate sleep problems.

In Chapter 3, we considered some of the scientific support for exercise as a means to improve sleep, but more has to be said. In a 1997 study published in the *Journal of the American Medical Association* (JAMA), scientists from Stanford University evaluated the effects of endurance exercise on forty-three sedentary but healthy adults, aged fifty to seventy-six. Their complaints included taking longer than twenty-five minutes to fall asleep and waking up after only six hours of sleep.

As a treatment, half of the group engaged in sixteen weeks of aerobic exercise. This included a weekly regimen of two one-hour, low-impact aerobic classes, plus two forty-minute sessions of brisk walking or stationary cycling. The other half of participants in the study did no exercise.

At the end of the investigation, those who had exercised said that they went to sleep about fifteen minutes sooner and slept about forty-five minutes longer than they had before beginning the exercise routine. In contrast, those who didn't exercise showed little or no improvement. (See *The New York Times,* January 1, 1997, p. 32.)

• Aerobic exercise and weight training can overcome stiffness, which may be associated with stress.

A generalized stiffness or physical creakiness is a common complaint among those who are under considerable negative stress. For older people, these complaints may arise from a link between stress and discomfort from the natural wear and tear on the joints from osteoarthritis.

In another 1997 study, also published in the January 1 issue of the *Journal of the American Medical Association,* researchers from the Bowman Gray School of Medicine in Winston-Salem, North Carolina, directed people with osteoarthritis to walk vigorously or work out with weights for three one-hour sessions per week. The investigators found that the exercisers experienced significant improvement in their body functions.

Specifically, the participants did a better job of climbing stairs, getting out of cars, and performing other daily activities. (Note: Such exercise is also recommended as a treatment for osteoarthritis by the Arthritis Foundation and the American College of Rheumatology.)

• Stretching is an effective treatment for stress.

A review article in *Patient Education and Counseling* (April 1994, pp. 5–12) surveyed the medical literature on stretching and relaxation training. The authors reported that stretch-based relaxation training (combining stretching with progressive relaxation of muscles) can have a significant effect in reducing muscle tension.

The studies cited in the review article show that tense patients have reported considerable improvement after using this approach. Electromagnetic measures of muscle tension showed greater physiologic relaxation. In particular, stretching and relaxation techniques, such as general meditation or focusing on the loosening of muscles, can assist in treatment of neck tension, various pains, and anxiety.

In a related observation, I'm reminded of the experience of one of my "stressed-out" patients who was a regular exerciser. He engaged in stretching and calisthenics about four mornings a week. Also, he pursued aerobic exercise, such as jogging and cycling, in the afternoons about four times a week.

In monitoring his responses during periods of heavy work and stress, the businessman reported that when he neglected his morning stretching—even when he was running or cycling regularly in the afternoons—he often suffered before lunch from a mildly stiff back and neck and a sense of "fuzzy-headedness." Yet when he did his stretches, he invariably felt fewer of these signs of stress in the morning.

• Weight and strength training can reduce overall stress on the body and improve physical functioning.

If you are under considerable stress *and* your muscles are generally out of shape, your ability to respond to unusual physical challenges—such as weekend exercise with a younger relative or even a long walk with friends—will be severely limited. On the other hand, if you cultivate above-average levels of muscle strength and stamina, your capacity to function physically at a high level can improve dramatically. The secret is to include strength training in your exercise program.

In a 1996 study conducted by the University of Vermont College of Medicine and the Mayo Clinic, and reported on April 15, 1996, in *The Washington Post*, researchers found that resistance training improved the walking endurance of twenty-four healthy but sedentary men and women, aged sixty-five to seventy-nine. Specifically, the participants not only gained in muscle strength and stamina, but also had to exert less effort to make it through a given walking time or distance. According to the researchers, the improvements were linked to the fact that the stress on the participants' bodies from the aerobic exercise was reduced through their increased strength.

Here's the way this study was set up:

The investigators divided the participants into two groups, with one group getting no exercise training, and the other being assigned to twelve weeks of resistance training (with exercise equipment), including leg extensions, leg curls, bench presses, and squats.

The group that did the exercises improved mobility and walking stamina significantly, according to measurements done during treadmill testing. But the physical capacities of the sedentary participants stayed about the same.

Before the study, the exercise group could walk an average of twenty-five minutes before fatigue forced them to stop. After the twelve-week exercise program, their performance time increased to an average of thirty-four minutes.

Another sign of excessive stress may be loss of bodily control and a tendency to experience more injuries through accidents, including falling or tripping. Yet in a study published on May 3, 1995, in the *Journal of the American Medical Association,* researchers found that regular exercise—including weight training, stretching, endurance training, and balance training—can reduce the incidence of falls by older people.

About 30 percent of people over age sixty-five fall at least once a year. Furthermore, 10 to 15 percent of those falls cause fractures of the hip or other bones, with a significant proportion of them resulting in death or permanent disability.

Yet the study found that regular exercise of any type could on average reduce the risk of falling by about 13 percent. Participants who engaged in the Chinese martial art of Tai Chi, which focuses on movements that require balance, showed a 25 percent reduction in their fall rate.

Of course, exercise, including aerobic exercise, has its limits as an antidote to stress and stress-related problems. If you push your body too hard—either by engaging in a short work-out that is too intense or by exercising too often or for too long—your exercise prescription may backfire. You can *increase* your susceptibility to the effects of bad stress.

Some of my recent books, including *Antioxidant Revolution* and *Faith-Based Fitness,* both published by Thomas Nelson, have provided extensive treatments of the dangers of excessive exercise. One of the greatest threats is that overdoing it may release too many free radicals in your body. These unstable oxygen molecules have been associated with more than fifty serious diseases, including heart problems, various cancers, and cataracts. Similarly, the free radicals released by doing too much strength work or unaccustomed stretching may cause sore, inflamed, and injured tissues.

One way to fight the negative effects of free radicals, including those produced by bad stress, is to increase your intake of antioxidants, especially vitamin E, vitamin C, and beta-carotene. (For recommendations on amounts of these antioxidants, see my *Antioxidant Revolution* and my *Advanced Nutritional Therapies,* both published by Thomas Nelson.)

Another way to counter the threat of free radicals is to limit the amount of exercise. The ultimate objective is to strike just the right balance: Your exercise should be intense enough to provide you with plenty of protection against bad stress, yet not so intense as to release free radicals.

Now let's move on to the practical question that begs to be answered: Exactly how much aerobic exercise is enough to give you the emotional and physical benefits you need without unnecessarily increasing your health risks?

Exactly How Much Aerobic Exercise Is Enough?

During the past thirty years, there has been a dramatic change in our understanding of the relationship of physical fitness to mental and physical health.

Through the 1970s and 1980s, I believed, as did most other preventive medicine experts, that the best way to be healthy—to reach a state of overall optimum well-being—was to achieve "aerobic fitness." If you wanted to derive any health benefits from exercise, you had to work out enough to produce an "aerobic training effect." This effect is based on continuous athletic activity for a certain period each week at an intensity that is within your "target heart rate" zone.

To calculate target heart rate, we have recommended using this formula: Begin with the figure 220 and subtract your age in years. This will give you your predicted maximal heart rate in beats per minute. Then, you proceed to find your target heart rate, which would be 65 to 80 percent of this predicted maximal heart rate. To achieve aerobic fitness, the goal is to exercise at this target heart rate for at least twenty minutes four times per week, or thirty minutes three times per week.

For example, a forty-five-year-old would go through these calculations: Subtract 45 (the age) from 220 to get 175, or the predicted maximal heart rate. Then, multiply this figure by 0.65 and 0.80 (65 percent and 80 percent) to get the target heart rate zone or range. This would mean a target heart rate of 114 to 140 beats per minute. Similarly, using the same formula, a fifty-five-year-old would have a target heart rate zone of 107 to 132 beats per minute.

These target heart rate zones are the ranges in which a person should exercise if he or she wants to achieve aerobic fitness—or a minimum level of athletic conditioning. But this way of thinking about fitness changed abruptly in November 1989 with the publication of a study in the *Journal of the American Medical Association* (pp. 2395–401) by Dr. Steven Blair of our Cooper Institute for Aerobics Research.

An Exercise Revolution

Up to the time of this *JAMA* report, we believed that the relatively high, aerobic level of fitness was essential for all purposes, including preparation for athletic performance or competition and optimum health and longevity. But Dr. Blair's report, which has been acclaimed generally by experts in preventive medicine as the "landmark study of the century" for exercise, points us in an entirely different direction.

Dr. Blair's investigation established three categories of fitness: (1) a sedentary or unconditioned state; (2) health and longevity fitness; and (3) aerobic fitness. His revolutionary conclusion was that you *didn't* have to reach the highest level of conditioning to be optimally healthy (though you might want to be at that level for athletic performance). Instead, all that was necessary was to reach the middle level of physical conditioning, or health and longevity fitness.

Here is how Dr. Blair reached his startling new conclusions: First, he followed 10,244 healthy men and 3,120 healthy women for slightly more than eight years. Then, he came up with his three fitness categories by measuring physical fitness according to the time the participants performed on a standardized treadmill stress test.

After the data were put through a computer analysis, with adjustments made for sex and age, Dr. Blair set up these categories:

- Those in the bottom 20th percentile of fitness were classified as "sedentary."
- The next 40 percent were classified as being in the "health and longevity fitness" category.
- The top 40 percent were the "aerobically fit" group.

This comprehensive research, which involved 110,482 "person years" of follow-up evaluations, showed that there was an average 58 percent reduction in deaths from all causes when people moved up from the sedentary category to the health and longevity category. Also, there was a slightly higher (65 percent) reduction between the sedentary category and the aerobic category.

What practical conclusions can we draw from Dr. Blair's findings?

The most important is that using his three-category system, the best "return" on your fitness "investment" involves not going from the lowest (sedentary) category to the highest (aerobic fitness) category. Rather, you get a better return from your energy and time expenditure by going from the sedentary category to the middle category of health and longevity fitness (which included those who were in the 20th to 60th percentile of fitness).

It's true, of course, that there is *slightly* more benefit if you reach the top category of fitness (a 65 percent reduction in deaths versus a 58 percent reduction). But overall, the health and longevity benefits tend to level off as your fitness increases.

Dr. Blair's new recommendations were well received by the scientific community and were included in the 1996 *Surgeon General's Report on Physical Activity and Health*. In fact, Dr. Blair was the senior editor of that report. Overall, the report provided a realistic way for the average, nonathletic person to receive significant benefits from exercise, but without the high demands placed on the trained athlete.

Subsequent studies from the Cooper Institute for Aerobics Research have confirmed and extended Dr. Blair's initial findings. In 1995, Dr. Blair and other researchers reported that even men who don't start their fitness programs until after age sixty are less likely than unfit men to die from all causes, including cardiovascular disease. (See *JAMA*, April 12, 1995, pp. 1093–8.) The next year, an investigation by our researchers determined that being totally sedentary carries an even greater risk of dying from all causes than does smoking one package of cigarettes per day! (See *JAMA*, July 17, 1996, pp. 205–10.)

Despite these research breakthroughs, some question has remained about *exactly how much* exercise is enough to provide significant health benefits, including relief from stress. For example, the Harvard Alumni Health Study concluded that "vigorous activities" are associated with longevity, while "nonvigorous activities" are not. (See *JAMA*, April 19, 1995, pp. 1179–84.)

The message of this study—which has been subject to some criticism because it is based on subjective participant questionnaires rather than on actual fitness testing—turns on the definitions of *vigorous* and *nonvigorous*. Some of the vigorous activities listed by the researchers included brisk walking, running, jogging, swimming laps, playing tennis, and shoveling snow.

According to standards set by the Harvard Alumni researchers, these activities had to be done often enough to burn up at least 1,500 calories per week. Translated into an actual workout, the type of exercise that could lead to a longer life might involve one of the following:

- Walking three miles in forty-five minutes or less, five times per week
- Swimming 1,200 yards in less than thirty minutes, three times per week
- Jogging three miles in less than thirty minutes, three times per week

In terms of my own system of aerobic points—and Dr. Blair's categories—this level of exercise would put a person at the high end of the middle (health and longevity fitness) category, or at the low end of the highest (aerobic fitness) category. So even though there may be some question about the reliability of the design of the Harvard study, the results are close to what we found in the Cooper Institute investigations.

To add to the uncertainty about how much exercise is necessary for you to combat stress effectively, let me mention yet another fitness paradox: We now know that you can be aerobically fit but also unhealthy.

Look at the case of the running guru Jim Fixx, who died in 1984 during a training run in the hills of Vermont. He was running up to sixty miles per week at the time of his death at age fifty-two and had covered an estimated 37,000 miles in seventeen years, including twenty marathons.

But the autopsy, which was conducted just after he died at the end of a four-mile run, revealed very advanced three-vessel coronary artery disease. The autopsy showed that he had suffered two previously undiagnosed heart attacks. So despite his high level of aerobic fitness, Fixx was quite unhealthy.

As I discussed in my *Running Without Fear* (Bantam, 1985), there were several possible reasons for Jim Fixx's untimely death. One was a family history of early cardiovascular disease. For example, his father, Calvin, suffered a massive heart attack when he was thirty-six and died of another heart attack at age forty-three. Another factor was Jim Fixx's failure to get regular medical exams, including stress tests. These checkups could have detected his problem and might have enabled him to prolong his life. Also, Fixx had an enlarged heart and probably a heart murmur, conditions that increased his risk of heart trouble.

An additional possibility that has come to my attention since the publication of *Running Without Fear* is that Fixx's intense exercise regimen may have contributed to his death. His demanding workouts may have actually increased the stress on his system to the danger point by producing too many destructive free radicals. These unstable oxygen molecules could have hastened the buildup of plaque in the coronary arteries.

Furthermore, because of his demanding personal responsibilities and professional schedule as a best-selling author and speaker, Fixx was exposed to considerable bad emotional stress. On at least one occasion, as he was about to do a television talk show in Chicago, he suffered a major anxiety attack with a wildly pounding heart and dizziness. The incident was so serious, he had to ask the interviewer to terminate the TV appearance.

From such reports it seems clear that Jim Fixx, despite his good physical condition, lacked adequate coping mechanisms to handle the stress in his life. In fact, his intense focus on his physical conditioning and his status as a competitive middle-aged athlete may well have backfired: Such a high-strung approach to exercise may *increase* the stress in one's life rather than function as an antidote to stress. Remember: Negative stress of all types—whether combined with physical activity or not—may produce extra free radicals, which have been linked to heart disease and other unhealthy changes in the body.

To sum up, then, the evidence shows that for general health benefits, it's necessary to stop being sedentary. But it's not necessary to become a superathlete. Working out too hard—or trying for too much "pain"—may impair your health and well-being.

The latest scientific findings suggest that the same principles of moderation apply to the use of exercise for stress management. In other words, more exercise is not necessarily better for your stress.

Consider a 1994 study conducted by scientists at Western Kentucky University, where they focused on the effect that *reducing* exercise levels can have on moods and emotions, including anxiety and depression. They divided fifty-seven heavy exercisers into three groups and placed them on these ten-week programs:

1. A control group continued to maintain their same intense exercise regimen.
2. A second group of heavy exercisers reduced their workouts to no more than five hours of moderate aerobic activity per week.
3. A third group maintained their current, heavy regimen, but also attended five one-and-one-half-hour relaxation training sessions.

The results: There was no statistically significant difference among any of the groups when they were tested as to their mood states, including anxiety and depression. In other words, moderate exercise is as good as heavy exercise in overcoming negative emotions, including the effects of bad stress. (See *Perceptions and Motor Skills,* December 1994, pp. 1635–44.)

My conclusion from all these studies and findings is this: If you want the best "return" on your exercise investment—in terms of general health, greater longevity, and stress management—focus on moderate (or in Dr. Blair's terms, "health and longevity fitness") exercise, as described earlier in this chapter. Doing less or more may hurt you.

Now, before we end this general discussion of exercise and health, let me offer some final words about a large group who merit special attention: I'm referring to women, and especially those who are under stress.

The Potential of the Exercise Prescription for Women Under Stress

First, the bad news: According to the Centers for Disease Control and Prevention (CDCP), almost three-fourths of American women are still not getting enough exercise. In particular, 73 percent of women eighteen years old and older do not meet the minimum aerobic requirements of twenty minutes per day, three days per week, of continuous endurance activity. This might involve brisk walking, jogging, or swimming. These women do not even engage in enough less strenuous activity, such as raking leaves or walking slowly at least thirty minutes per day, five days per week.

Older women are the most likely to be sedentary, with 42 percent of those sixty-five and older being totally inactive, as compared with 26 percent of those eighteen to thirty-four.

Teenage girls are among the most chronic couch potatoes, according to the CDCP: Only 37 percent of female students in grades ten through twelve exercise vigorously—a figure that is down from 68 percent in 1984.

Despite these gloomy statistics, there is a bright side to the exercise picture for women. First of all, the general benefits that men enjoy are also available to women. For example, a 1995 presentation at the American Heart Association's annual epidemiology meeting in San Antonio reported on a Harvard Medical School study on the exercise habits of more than 73,000 women. This investigation found that those who were most active had about a 40 percent lower risk of heart attacks and strokes than the least active. The active women in the study had a major advantage even when only moderate levels of exercise were involved.

But perhaps the best evidence of the positive potential of exercise on health—and especially on stress—is to take a brief peek at what regular workouts can accomplish in the life of one busy woman who is constantly exposed to the pressures of life.

The following account, which has been edited only slightly for this discussion, was mailed to me in 1993 by Sue McElyea, who is a wife, the mother of three, and a full-time career professional. She sent a picture with her letter, and from her excellent condition and obviously brimming health, I assumed that she was in her early thirties until I read on and found that her *oldest child* was close to thirty! Here is her story in her own words, which began in the mid-seventies when her children were still at home and her career was in full swing.

One Woman's Triumph over the Stresses of Life: The Sue McElyea Story

My husband had been jogging for about three months, and he encouraged me to join him at our local high school track in Conyers, Georgia. All my life I had experienced weak ankles, a result of rheumatic fever as a child. I really never thought running was something I could endure.

My first run at the track was exactly one-fourth of one lap, which equates to approximately one-sixteenth of a mile. I was winded and could not keep going. However, never being one to quit, I was determined to improve.

Each day, I targeted more and more distance to conquer. Finally, I could run one mile without stopping, then two, then three, then four, five, and six. Four months later, by Labor Day, I entered a race at the insistence of a friend, who was my doctor. I had just turned thirty years old, and so I qualified to run in the thirty to forty age category. To my amazement, I won!

But that was my first and last race because running competitively interfered with my tennis. I can only play on weekends, and that is when most races are scheduled.

Even though I couldn't compete in races, I continued running every day, and on May 1, 1977, I began keeping a record of my workouts. Since that day, I have not missed one day of running. During the past twenty years I have traveled a great deal for work and pleasure, but I run wherever I happen to be:

Central Park, Hyde Park, various cities in Germany, Hawaii, cruise ships, trains, hotel parking garages, hotel roofs, or interstate rest areas. Most of my jogging takes place around San Antonio, Texas, where we have lived for the past eighteen years.

I run twice a day, one hour in the morning and one-half hour at night, in all weather conditions. Occasionally, I have missed my night run because of flights or appointments, but I have not missed my morning run in more than twenty years.

How far do I typically go during a workout? I'm not sure because I run for time rather than distance. It's hard to determine exactly the miles I have accumulated, but I estimate I have covered approximately sixty thousand miles since I started.

Using your books as guides, my husband and I have patterned our programs after your suggestions. We have also encouraged our children to run—and they all do. I personally feel very strongly that I would not be in nearly as good health as I am if it were not for my jogging. If you ever need someone for a study on the long-term effects of aerobic exercise, I could will my body for research, but I hope this won't be for a long time.

• • • •

The cheerful tone of the correspondence I have had with Sue makes it clear to me that despite her busy life, with unusual pressures of family and career constantly bearing down, she manages her stress well. Any negative stress in her life seems to have been transformed into positive stress—largely through her experience with aerobic exercise.

So let me leave you with these thoughts:

- Consider how packed Sue's life is now, and compare your own schedule. See if you have any more pressures than she has confronted.
- Remember how she started off in a totally unfit, low-energy condition—but in only four months became a winning, competitive athlete!
- Consider the tone of her letter, including the sense of satisfaction with life and the apparent mastery she possesses over stress.
- Finally, allow yourself to draw inspiration from her steady, consistent commitment to her exercise regimen.

I'm certainly not saying that you should go out and try to become a master athlete, or that you should work out two times a day, seven days a week, as Sue does. For most people—including me—that level of exercise is just not feasible or advisable. As this chapter makes abundantly clear, you don't have to go nearly that far with your program to get significant health and stress-reduction benefits.

But a person like Sue McElyea can at least serve as a model of what is possible for those who are concerned about managing the stress in their lives better—and who finally decide, "Yes, I do want to take advantage of nature's best tranquilizer."

But as important a weapon as exercise can be in fighting stress, a complete antistress program requires us to go still deeper—all the way down to the chemical and molecular levels that serve as the very foundations of our physical beings.

CHAPTER 5

UNVEILING THE MYSTERY OF MOLECULAR BALANCE

Where do you stand in writing your own Paradox Prescription against stress? At this point, you have finished the first three steps in your program to "immunize" yourself against bad stress:

First, in Chapter 3, you learned about the importance of a paradoxical mind-set or perspective on life.

Second, you were introduced in Chapter 3 to the tremendous importance of sleep in stress management.

Third, we explored in Chapter 4 the benefits of various types of exercise in improving your physical and emotional health, including your ability to handle stress.

Now, you are ready to consider Step #4 in your Paradox Prescription: learning to fight bad stress on the molecular level.

At first glance, taking our discussion down to chemical and molecular interactions may seem too abstract and impractical. But I assure you, the opposite is true. This chapter involves some of the most down-to-earth information you'll encounter in this book.

The molecular mystery of stress presents us with another paradox: The unseen, unfelt forces in our bodies may seem insignificant, but they are by far among the most important factors that determine health and longevity. Consider the following brief scenario depicting some of the potential for molecular chaos to get an idea about what an impact stress can have on you.

A Trigger for Molecular Madness

Bad stress can be a trigger for what I call "molecular madness"—or a dangerous disturbance in the delicate balance of hormones, chemicals, and other microcomponents deep inside our bodies. We often won't feel anything when such an imbalance occurs—at least not at first. But over time, molecular madness can maim and even kill.

Specifically, stress may produce this inner turmoil in at least six major "scenes," or areas: (1) adrenal hormones; (2) free radicals; (3) cholesterol levels; (4) the immune system; (5) blood glucose; and indirectly, (6) the buildup of bone mass. Here are the details.

Scene #1: The Fight-or-Flight Hormones

In Chapter 2, we examined the impact on the mind and body of the hormones produced under stress by the two adrenal glands. As you know, these glands, which are situated near the kidneys in the upper, back part of the abdominal cavity, produce such hormones as adrenaline (epinephrine), noradrenaline (norepinephrine), and cortisol. All of these substances prepare the body to respond physically to stressors. But problems arise if there is no physical outlet for these hormones. They may build up and cause permanent, negative changes (or adaptations) in the body, such as elevated blood pressure.

We have already considered commonplace stresses and strains—such as those that occur in a high-pressure work situation, automobile traffic, or jury duty—which may cause the release of adrenal hormones. But another, more dramatic adrenal connection to stress, which has received attention in recent years among scientists, involves the changes that may occur in the human body and emotions during and after natural catastrophes.

For example, terrifying events such as earthquakes and hurricanes can result in such serious stress-related responses as heart attacks and suicide. Scientists at the Good Samaritan Hospital in Los Angeles studied death records associated with the 1994 Los Angeles earthquake. They found that the number of deaths from heart attacks on January 17, 1994, the day the Northridge earthquake hit, was five times above normal expectations. But in the six days following the quake, heart attack deaths dipped below the average.

According to a report published in the *New England Journal of Medicine* on February 15, 1996, this sharp rise in deaths, followed by a decrease, indicates that the quake triggered deaths among those who were at particularly high risk of dying during the week that the disaster struck. In effect, those who were on the verge of a heart attack died earlier than they would have if the quake had not hit. Related research connected with this study suggested that 41 percent of all sudden cardiac deaths were due to a stressful event. (See *The New York Times*, February 15, 1996, p. A10.)

Scientists have speculated that the internal mechanism that produces heart attacks during an earthquake is a sudden release of adrenaline into the bloodstream, which increases the heart rate and blood flow. These changes may cause the heart to begin an unorganized quivering, so that the pumping action is interrupted; they may loosen plaque in the arteries to form a deadly blockage; or these changes may impede blood flow by creating spasms in an artery. (See *The Miami Herald*, February 15, 1996, p. 1A.)

Deaths during or after a hurricane disaster are more difficult to evaluate. One reason is that, unlike what happens with an earthquake, there is always a warning of several days before a hurricane hits. This delay tends to prevent the sudden release of adrenal hormones that occurs during an unanticipated earthquake.

Researchers in the study cited in *The Miami Herald* noted that heart attacks did occur during Hurricane Andrew in

Florida in 1992, but many of them were linked to events indirectly related to the high winds. For example, some people had heart attacks when they saw their destroyed property after the storm or when they were trying to clear out the debris.

Another variation on this stress-and-disaster theme is that health workers have found that suicide rates may go up in the days and months following a particularly devastating earthquake. The January 1995 quake in Kobe, Japan, is an illustration. Nurses and psychologists interviewed in the nine months following that disaster reported sharp rises in alcoholism, mental illness (especially depression), and suicide. (See *The Washington Post* report published in *The Miami Herald,* October 9, 1995, p. 7A.)

A possible scientific explanation for the increased incidence of suicides after natural disasters has emerged in a report in the *Journal of Child Psychology.* (See the May 1996 issue, pp. 435–44.) This study, conducted by researchers from the Department of Sociology, University of Miami, Coral Gables, pinpointed stress, among other influences, as an important risk factor for suicides after Hurricane Andrew. Other characteristics of persons committing suicide included being female, having low socioeconomic status, suffering depression, and exhibiting a prehurricane tendency toward suicide.

This link of stress to postdisaster suicide rates suggests that there may be lingering, unhealthful effects of adrenal hormones long after any initial burst of adrenaline. The bad stress—and initial output from the adrenal glands—begins with worry about the impending hurricane. The anxiety rises during the disaster and then continues for months afterward as victims try to pick up the pieces of their lives. The accompanying chemical changes in the body may have quite serious, and even deadly, effects on moods and emotions.

A related problem that has become the focus of many news reports in recent years involves stresses that occur during and after wartime experiences. The symptoms, which have been similar following most major wars during the past century and a half, include fatigue, shortness of breath, headaches, muscle and joint pains, sleep disturbances, and problems with concentration and memory. (See *The Wall Street Journal,* January 6, 1997, p. A14.) As you can see, these symptoms are practically identical to the general symptoms that I listed for bad stress in Chapter 2.

The wartime malady has gone under various names. In the Civil War, it was "irritable heart"; in World War I, "effort syndrome"; in World War II, "combat stress reaction"; in the Vietnam War, "post-traumatic stress disorder"; and in the 1992 Gulf War, "Gulf War syndrome."

A concern with the Gulf War syndrome was that the root of the problem may have been exposure to chemicals on the battlefield. But the symptoms cited still bear an eerie likeness to those of stress-related problems among veterans of other wars. Again, the release of fight-or-flight adrenal hormones may have been a factor in the deterioration of health.

Scene #2: Free Radicals

Stressful influences may also cause physical damage through the release of excess free radicals. (See my *Antioxidant Revolution.*)

A report in the July 1993 issue of *Epidemiology* focused on the impact of stressful events on more than one thousand Swedish patients. The researchers found that serious stress on the job caused a person to be five times as likely to get cancer of the colon or rectum. The reason is, apparently, as we know from other research, that free radicals may damage the DNA of the body's cells, a process that can lead to cancer.

Furthermore, these scientists found that patients who were unemployed longer than six months had twice the risk of cancer, and those who moved more than 120 miles had three times the risk. Going through a divorce or suffering the death of a spouse increased the person's cancer risk by 50 percent.

The Swedish scientists were unable to ascertain the exact cause of these serious health problems. But clearly, there was a link between stressful influences and cancer. The best interpretation at this point seems to be the involvement of excess free radicals released by the bad stress during crises.

Scene #3: Cholesterol

We have known for a long time that high total cholesterol is an important risk factor for cardiovascular disease, including clogging of the arteries (atherosclerosis) and heart attacks. As the research has accumulated over the years, high stress has emerged as a factor that may be linked to high cholesterol. (See "Cholesterol, Stress, Lifestyle, and Coronary Heart Disease," *Aviation, Space, and Environmental Medicine,* July 1985.)

Specifically, we have learned these facts:

- In a study of medical students with high cholesterol at Johns Hopkins Medical School, participants who suffered heart attacks at an early age also were identified as being unusually sensitive to stress. (See *Johns Hopkins Medical Journal,* 1975, vol. 136, pp. 193–208.)
- Norwegian medical students experienced a 20 percent increase in their total cholesterol during a very important academic examination. (See *Experimental and Clinical Endocrinology,* 1984, vol. 83, no. 3, pp. 361–3.)
- Other studies have shown that total cholesterol levels go up significantly when men lose their jobs, when students in navy underwater demolition (UDT) programs are in the final weeks of training, and when surgery patients are about to have their operations. (See my *Controlling Cholesterol* [Bantam, 1989], pp. 288ff.)

Scene #4: The Immune Function

Stress can play a major role in the immune function, but the exact mechanisms may be more complicated than we have always thought.

The straightforward understanding is that stress depresses the immune function and thereby makes us more vulnerable to various diseases. There have been many reports of immune-related diseases or reactions during or after a stressful influence.

For example, Dr. Miguel R. Sanchez, a dermatologist at the New York University School of Medicine, has reported an increase in canker sores in the mouth when a person is under stress—whether the stress is physical, emotional, or chemical. These often develop right before a cold or during a period of excessive fatigue. (See release, New York University Medical Center, April 10, 1995.)

Investigators at the Harry S. Truman Memorial Veterans Hospital, Columbia, Missouri, have established that stress-management training results in statistically significant relief from many symptoms of rheumatoid arthritis. Patients in this study showed improvement in their sense of helplessness, self-esteem, coping ability, pain, and general health. (See *Arthritis and Rheumatology,* December 1995, pp. 1807–18.)

Note: Although the exact causes of rheumatoid arthritis are not clear, many experts believe that this disease arises from immune-related genetic problems.

The link between stress and immunity has grown cloudier, however, as a result of recent research, including investigations by two neuroscientists from Rockefeller University in New York, Dr. Bruce McEwen and Firdaus S. Dhabhar, a doctoral candidate. In 1995, they reported both in the *Journal of Immunology* and in oral presentations that mild stress will not reduce the body's immune cells. Rather, this type of pressure will cause the immune cells, such as killer cells and special white blood cells, to be redistributed to the site of the stressful attack. In other words, mild stress doesn't make the immune system "crash"; instead, mild stress marshals it for a more effective response.

On the other hand, the researchers reported that *chronic* stress, which is applied to the body and mind over a long period of time, can actually suppress immune cells. (See *The New York Times*, November 21, 1995, p. B10.)

The lesson from these findings seems to be that the immune system functions as it was designed to function when stress hits initially. But if we fail to manage that stress well, our immune systems may become overloaded, and our vulnerability to immune-related diseases will increase.

Scene #5: Blood Sugar (Glucose)

Another "scene" in our bodies where stress can have a big impact is the bloodstream, where blood glucose or sugar is found. Researchers at the Department of Behavioral Medicine and Psychiatry, West Virginia University, evaluated the blood glucose, stress levels, and coping mechanisms in eight people with non-insulin-dependent diabetes. They found that blood sugar was significantly higher on high-stress days, as compared with low-stress days. Also, they discovered evidence of a relationship among stress, coping mechanisms, and blood sugar. (See *Behavioral Research and Therapy*, June 1994, pp. 503–10.)

Clearly, this study indicates that stress can be particularly dangerous for persons with a tendency toward diabetes or high blood sugar. In addition, people with diabetes who fail to develop good coping mechanisms for dealing with stress are placing themselves at higher risk.

An exercise connection is apparent. According to researchers, the subjects were significantly less active on high-stress days (when blood sugar was highest) than on low-stress days. This result suggests a paradox: People under stress simply don't make time for exercise, even though exercise is a "treatment" that could do them worlds of good. Furthermore, their failure to exercise may well have exacerbated their stressed-out condition and contributed to their high blood-sugar levels.

Scene #6: Bone Cells

The final "scene" in which the molecular madness of stress is being played out is the skeletal structure, but here, the effects of stress may be direct or indirect.

Paradoxically, by putting *physical* stress on the bones—that is, by doing weight-bearing exercise such as running or using barbells—you can make your skeletal structure stronger. This type of activity stimulates the "osteoblasts," or bone-building cells, to build up bone tissue faster than normal.

On the other hand, responding negatively to *emotional* stress can have the opposite effect on your bones. One *direct* way that the skeletal structure may be harmed by bad stress was highlighted during a 1996 conference in Washington, D.C., which was sponsored by the International Society for Neuroimmunomodulation. At a November 15 meeting, Dr. Philip Gold of the National Institute of Mental Health said that the release of adrenal hormones, such as cortisol, can destroy appetite, impair the immune system, interrupt the repair of bodily tissue, disrupt sleep, and even contribute to a loss of bone mass.

To support his claim, Dr. Gold presented a study that had evaluated the bone density of twenty-six women, all of whom were forty years of age. Half of them were depressed, and the other half were emotionally normal. He reported that the depressed women had high levels of stress hormones and that they had bone density measurements comparable to those of seventy-year-old women. (See Associated Press release, published November 17, 1996.)

Some other ways of responding to bad stress may have an *indirect* effect in hindering bone growth and maintenance. These responses include smoking, drinking too much alcohol, taking in extra coffee and other caffeine-laced drinks, developing eating disorders, and experiencing an upset stomach and lowered appetite. Each of these responses can work against developing strong bones.

Various medical studies have linked smoking and high caffeine and alcohol intake to bone diseases such as osteoporosis. For example, research has shown that cigarette smoking lowers women's estrogen levels, and those with low estrogen are at much higher risk for osteoporosis. As for alcohol, having more than a drink or two per day inhibits the formation of new bone-building activity in the body.

Research is still in a fairly preliminary stage on the impact of caffeine-containing drinks on bones. But currently, the best thinking is that you will increase your risk of bone loss and osteoporosis if you drink three or more cups of coffee per day, or the caffeine equivalent in other caffeine-containing drinks and colas.

Any factors that work against a good appetite—such as eating disorders or an upset stomach—will decrease the amount of calcium and other nutrients essential for bone development.

· · · ·

Stress may be triggering many disturbing events at the molecular level in your body. So don't be fooled just because you don't feel or see huge physical changes taking place. The subtle symptoms of bad stress mentioned in Chapter 2—including fatigue, headaches, backaches, upset stomachs, and the like—should be sufficient to alert you to the danger.

But even before you identify the signs or symptoms, you should take steps to minimize the chemical and hormonal effects of bad stress. To this end, review the following checklist for preventing molecular madness.

Prescriptions for Preventing Molecular Madness

Here are some suggestions that have been proven to work in decreasing or eliminating the negative effects of stress on your body. You have seen some of them before, and subsequent chapters will mention others or expand upon them. In any event, these "prescriptions" are highlighted at this point as effective ways to keep your body's invisible internal systems in a healthful balance.

First Prescription: Check Your Diet

Probably the most powerful way to avoid stress-produced molecular madness is to evaluate and adjust your eating habits.

Cholesterol control

Because stress may raise cholesterol levels, you should do everything you can to keep your cholesterol as low as possible. This way, if you experience a "cholesterol spike" with stress, the high point of your lipid (blood fat) measurements will tend to be lower than if your normal cholesterol reading begins at a high level.

The best dietary way to keep cholesterol low is to limit your intake of saturated fats, such as those found in butter, whole milk, and various meats. My recommendation is to limit your intake of all fats to no more than 30 percent, and preferably no more than 25 percent, of your total intake of calories every day. Of these fat calories, no more than one-third should come from saturated fats, with another third coming from monounsaturated fats (such as olive oil), and the final third from polyunsaturated fats (such as those in margarine and corn oil).

This means that if you consume 2,500 calories daily, your total intake of fats should not exceed 625 to 750 calories. Your intake of saturated fats should be limited to 208 to 250 calories.

To keep your cholesterol low through your diet, you should limit or avoid foods that are high in cholesterol, such as eggs and high-fat cheeses. The total intake of cholesterol for the average person without a problem with cholesterol should be no more than about 250 milligrams per day. In general, those with total cholesterol over 200 milligrams per deciliter should keep their cholesterol intake below 200 milligrams per day—and even lower if total cholesterol measurements are well above 200 mg/dl. (For specific recommendations, see my *Controlling Cholesterol* [Bantam, 1989], p. 53.)

Free radical control

Strong evidence suggests that you can be protected against the destruction of free radicals by increasing your intake of antioxidants in the diet and through supplements. The main antioxidants you should consume are vitamin C, vitamin E, and beta-carotene. My basic recommendations involve the daily intake of 400 international units (IU) of vitamin E, 500 to 1,000 milligrams of vitamin C, and 25,000 IU of beta-carotene.

The best way to get these vitamins is through the diet, but that's not always possible, especially with vitamin E. So feel free to take supplements to be sure you reach your daily quota. (For more specific recommendations on these nutrients, other antioxidants, and important supplements like folic acid, see my *Antioxidant Revolution* and my *Advanced Nutritional Therapies*, both published by Thomas Nelson.)

Although the consensus is that people should receive plenty of antioxidants through the diet, discussions continue to percolate in scientific studies about the extent to which supplements should be used. Increasingly, however, there is a movement toward recommending relatively large doses of supplements in the amounts I have suggested here.

For example, in one recent research effort reported in *The New York Times* (October 7, 1996, p. C2), Roc Ordman, the chairman of the biochemistry department of Beloit College in Wisconsin, reported that he had monitored fifty healthy adults to see how fast the body lost vitamin C. The adults studied included all ages, genders, and physical sizes, though none were obese.

Ordman found that with healthy adults, 500 milligrams of vitamin C taken twice a day in supplement form—or a total of 1,000 milligrams per day—were sufficient to keep the body well saturated. His support for a "saturation principle" is consistent with the belief of a growing number of scientists, who feel that the optimum dose for antioxidants should be set at a level that will keep the body's cells and tissues soaked. Lesser amounts may not provide full antioxidant benefits, but excessive amounts will be excreted.

Second Prescription: Remember Exercise

You've already been introduced in some depth in Chapter 4 to exercise as an antidote to stress. But here are some further reminders about the importance of exercise as a treatment for molecular madness.

Take cholesterol, for instance. In general, the higher your level of "good," HDL (high-density lipoprotein) cholesterol, the lower your cardiovascular risk. Aerobic exercise is the best *natural* way to raise HDL.

Moderate aerobic exercise may also be protective against the damage of free radicals. Your body has a natural defense system of internal chemicals—known as "endogenous antioxidants"—which work to neutralize destructive free radicals. These include enzymes with such mysterious designations as "SOD," "GSH," and "catalase." Although excessive exercise may produce extra free radicals that overwhelm these internal antioxidants, moderate or lower-intensity exercise seems to strengthen the internal system of protection.

For example, a 1993 report in *Medicine and Science in Sports and Medicine* investigated the life expectancy of more than 2,600 world-class Finnish athletes. The researchers found that the endurance athletes in the study who continued to exercise at a lower intensity after their competitive careers were finished had the greatest life expectancy of all. This result suggests that a lifetime program of moderate endurance exercise is an effective way to shore up the body's defenses against life-threatening diseases.

Third Prescription: Consider Medical Intervention

If your "stress checkup" described in Chapter 9 indicates you have a problem with cholesterol, blood glucose, or another area of body chemistry, medical intervention may be required.

If you have elevated or unbalanced cholesterol, your physician may suggest an over-the-counter drug, such as niacin. Niacin can lower "bad" (LDL) cholesterol and raise "good" (HDL) cholesterol. Or you may need a prescribed medication, such as Mevacor, Zocor, Pravachol, or Lipitor.

If you live in an earthquake-prone region—and your doctor suspects your cardiovascular system may be in danger from stress during such a natural disaster—he or she may prescribe a medication like aspirin or a beta-blocker. These can help prevent the closing of coronary vessels to the heart during a stress attack and thus may help prevent a heart attack. (See the February 15, 1996, *New England Journal of Medicine* article discussed earlier in the chapter.)

These are some of the main prescriptions that can quell the molecular madness that stress may cause in your body. But some highly effective responses to bad stress reach well beyond the physical and into the spiritual realm. This "mind-spirit challenge" to stress is our next topic for discussion.

CHAPTER 6

RISING TO THE MIND-SPIRIT CHALLENGE

Even though the worst damage may finally be done to the body, most bad stress enters the body through the mind.

Suppose you experience a death in the family, or a divorce, or extreme criticism from your boss at work. Or maybe you are subjected to an angry attack by an acquaintance. All these influences are stressors that must pass through your emotions and other mental processes before they can damage your body. None of them are able to launch a direct physical hit all by itself.

Stressors typically operate *first* on the mind. Then, the mind may pass on bad stress to the body in some unhealthful response, such as higher blood pressure, a faster heart rate, a headache, a backache, or an upset stomach.

But the mind does not have to become the servant of negative stress. It stands to reason that if the general events and circumstances of life can condition your mind and emotions to respond negatively to stressors, the opposite is also possible: Your mind can be trained to neutralize negative stress or to turn it into a positive, motivating force in your life. That's what Step #5 of the Paradox Prescription is all about—meeting and conquering the "mind-spirit challenge" posed by bad stress.

But before we move on in this discussion, a few definitions are in order: specifically, the medical and scientific meaning of words such as *mind* and *spirit.*

The Great Medical Debate over the Mind and the Spirit

First, let me say a few words about the meaning of the terms *mind* and *mental* as they are used in medical practice and research.

A vast body of scientific literature in the stress field goes under such names as "mind-body interactions," "mental therapy," or "mental healing." These are general designations for psychological strategies that work in treating stress problems and other emotional problems. Some of these techniques, which we'll discuss later in this chapter, include relaxation training, reminiscence, writing therapy, music therapy, humor, and what is often called "cognitive-behavioral therapy."

Although researchers acknowledge that many mental therapy approaches work, they can't always determine *why* they work. One reason for this uncertainty is that we don't really understand the relationship between what we call the mind to the physical neurons and synapses and other tissues that make up the brain.

A philosophical debate has been raging for years about whether the mind is a separate entity at all. The nagging question persists, Is the mind identical to the physical brain, or is it somehow different—and perhaps even transcendent?

Sir John Eccles, the winner of the Nobel Prize in medicine in 1963, has argued that the mind is *not* rooted in physical tissues and cells, but instead transcends biology. He has even said that he believes the mind, which is the key to human identity, is somehow "from a divine creation." (See Herbert Benson, *Your Maximum Mind* [New York: Times Books, 1987], p. 45.)

In general, Eccles's position has been supported by other scientists, including Wilder Penfield, the Canadian neurosurgeon. Penfield has said that the mind is independent of the brain and is the agent that "programs" the computerlike brain.

In opposition to this line of argument, the neurophysiologist William H. Calvin has argued in *How Brains Think* (New York: Basic Books, 1996) and elsewhere that our creative thoughts and consciousness—what we generally refer to as mind—have arisen through Darwinian, physical evolution.

Also, he suggests, our sense of self has developed not from some outside, divine origin, but from impressions made by countless life experiences on our hardwired cerebral biology.

In other words, as far as Calvin is concerned, mind isn't transcendent at all, nor does it have a divine source or dimension. Rather, he believes, mind is more an earthbound, physical phenomenon.

Once you affirm the mind as existing above or separate from the body, it's just a short step to accepting a spiritual realm of reality. Many scientists and physicians who research and prescribe stress therapy often blur the distinction between the mental realm and the spiritual realm. They move rather easily from relaxation training to cognitive therapy to prayer, depending on how they feel a patient will respond.

But what exactly do researchers mean when they use the term *spiritual?*

The Medical Meaning of Spiritual

Like most people, I have a personal religious orientation—in my case, a traditional Christian faith. In that context, my use of the term *spiritual* is rooted in the Bible and historic Old and New Testament theology.

But as a preventive medicine specialist, I have to deal with the spiritual label in a somewhat different way. The medical literature on treatments for stress and other emotional disturbances is filled with references to spiritual strategies and cures. But what do scientists and researchers mean when they use the term?

To provide a context for our discussion, I need to point out a couple of common understandings of the term. When no capital letter is used, *spirit* is assumed by most nontheologians—as well as most physicians and medical researchers—to refer to the vital, life-giving, divinely generated breath, spark, or principle that makes human beings distinctively human. (When a capital letter is used, *Spirit* usually means the "Holy Spirit.")

This understanding of *spirit* as a religiously based principle that goes beyond the physical world has a direct bearing on the medical use of the term. In particular, there has been an increasing tendency to describe certain religion-connected medical techniques for coping with stress as "spiritual."

For example, a July 1993 report in *Clinical Nurse Specialist* (pp. 175–82) noted a current trend in medical circles to use the term *spiritual* in a broad context. This usage includes treatments that in some way rely on traditional religious practice, a general belief in or acceptance of transcendence, and various relational interactions, including those in the nurse-patient and doctor-patient relationships.

After questioning nineteen surgery patients, twelve nurses, and seven chaplains, the researchers arrived at these conclusions about the meaning and use of the term *spiritual* in medical settings:

• Common spiritual needs of patients included their need for help and support in dealing with religion, values, relationships, beliefs in transcendence, various emotions and feelings, and problems in communication.

- The respondents also identified five common spiritual interventions or practices by nurses in their work with patients: praying; reading Scripture and discussing it; being present with a patient; listening to the patient; and referring patient concerns to experts in spiritual matters.

This research suggests that, from a medical viewpoint, there may be an overlap between mental and spiritual strategies. For example, emotional and relational concerns could easily fall into either category. But some practices and techniques, such as prayer and religious counseling, must be seen as distinctively spiritual.

Now, with this background in mind, let's consider practical stress-reduction strategies involving the mind and the spirit. Some of these techniques should be helpful as you try to manage the bad stress in your life. First, we'll focus on therapies dealing primarily with the mind.

Freeing Your Shackled Mind

When you are under heavy pressure, your mind may in effect be shackled by stress. You may be so preoccupied with a particular concern or worry that you are unable to concentrate productively on your work or important relationships. Or you may be in a constant state of irritation, anger, or fear because of a personal or family crisis.

These emotional "prisons" can be minimized or eliminated with one or more of the following mental techniques, which researchers have found effective in freeing the mind from stress.

Cognitive-Behavioral Therapy

This technical-sounding term is a catchall for several rather straightforward and well-established psychological techniques for overcoming bad stress. In general, the idea is to change your usual way of thinking and acting so that your feelings of being stressed out are changed or eradicated.

Specifically, with cognitive-behavioral therapy you may learn to relabel your stress problem (or stressor) so that you can approach it in a more productive way.

Suppose, for instance, that you are worried because your adult son can't make up his mind about a career, and you have decided he is "mixed up," "indecisive," or just "inept." You feel you know what's wrong with him, and you have a plan for him to redirect his life, but he won't listen to you. No matter how hard you try, you can't control him.

This attitude causes you to worry constantly. You continue to contact your son and attempt to persuade him to follow your advice, but you don't get to first base. As a result, you lose sleep, experience physical aches and pains, frequently have an upset stomach, and display other signs of stress.

You may find your way out of this emotional prison if you relabel the problem: You may decide that your son is going through a normal phase for some young adults. Or perhaps you could describe his problems as "developmental" and accept the idea that eventually, he will "outgrow" his lack of career focus.

Of course, relabeling won't work unless there is a factual or rational justification for it. But most worries of this type are subject to more than one interpretation. Relabeling is a way for you to see the situation from another angle and in the process lower your levels of bad stress.

Another effective cognitive-behavioral approach is to *explain to yourself* why you are feeling stressed out. As you go through this exercise, identify your specific stressors, and examine them in detail to see why they are such a powerful influence in your life. Also, analyze the stressors in terms of how likely they are to last and what you might do to get rid of them.

Still another way to reduce the power of bad stress is to *employ a distraction or substitution technique.* In brief, this means taking steps to turn your attention away from the stressor, sometimes by substituting another thought or activity to occupy your thinking. It's best if the substitute activity you choose has the power in itself to capture your interest or concentration instead of requiring you to supply the mental initiative or horsepower.

For example, to break a "stress tape" that keeps running over and over in your mind, such as worry over a personal financial matter, you might go out and take a walk, jog, or play tennis. Or if you're not feeling particularly athletic, you could turn on some music or see a movie or play.

Typically, therapists find that such distractions or substitute activities don't have to be pursued for very long to be effective. As little as fifteen minutes may be enough to ease the sense of stress. On the other hand, an activity like reading a difficult novel or book of philosophy might not provide an antidote to your stress no matter how long you keep at it because such activities require extra mental effort and concentration.

How well do these techniques work? Many scientific studies proclaim the effectiveness of cognitive-behavioral therapy in treating stress. For example, researchers at the Department of Psychology, University of Houston, reporting in a 1994 study published in the *Journal of Consulting Clinical Psychology*, found that cognitive-behavioral therapy helped significantly with panic disorders and various fears, including agoraphobia (fear of leaving home and entering open public places). (See the August 1994 issue, pp. 818–26.)

Similarly, in a 1995 study conducted by the Department of Psychology, University of New South Wales, Australia, investigators reviewed the literature on the impact of cognitive-behavioral therapy on generalized anxiety disorder (GAD). They determined that this type of therapy may provide a long-term and cost-effective solution to GAD patients, who typically say they have "always been worriers."

Other research has demonstrated that cognitive-behavioral therapies can produce physical changes in the biology of the brain. In a study published in the *Archives of General Psychiatry* (February 15, 1996), PET scans were done on patients with obsessive-compulsive disorder before and after ten weeks of cognitive-behavioral therapy. They showed significant changes in brain functioning, including an alteration in physical connections and in signals emitted in specific parts of the brain, such as the caudate nucleus, the cingulate gyrus, and the thalamus. (See *The New York Times*, February 15, 1996, p. C22.)

But cognitive-behavioral therapy is only one among many possibilities for the mental or psychological regulation of stress. Another category involves several strategies that may be grouped under the general umbrella of "relaxation training."

Relaxation Training

Many types of relaxation training can be used to prevent bad stress reactions. But the most effective types seem to have one thing in common: They elicit what has been designated as the "relaxation response"—a concept identified in the early 1970s by Dr. Herbert Benson of the Harvard Medical School.

This physiologic response, which has become a standard term in stress treatment literature, is defined in *Stedman's Medical Dictionary* and other medical references as an "integrated reaction" in the part of the brain known as the "hypothalamus" (located just below the cerebrum, or higher brain center). Accompanying physical changes may include lower heart rate, lower blood pressure, and a generalized feeling of being stress-free.

Stedman's Medical Dictionary notes that the relaxation response is almost a "mirror image"—or the exact opposite—

of the body's fight-or-flight responses while under stress. Obviously, if you experience symptoms of bad stress, doing what you can to elicit the relaxation response is highly desirable.

A number of relaxation techniques may trigger this physical reaction:

• Simple muscle-relaxing exercises

One classic approach is to focus mentally on your toes and feet. As you focus, practice tightening the muscles throughout your feet and then relaxing them. When the tension has left your feet, move to the muscles in your lower legs, and repeat the exercise. Move up through your whole body in this way. By the time you get to your forehead, your stress level should be much lower.

• Simple meditation

As Dr. Benson has emphasized throughout his books and articles, the type of meditation that he advocates—and has tested scientifically—is a generic technique. That is, it's *not* tied to a particular religious system. But interestingly enough, in his clinical work Benson has found that the approach works best when used with one's personal beliefs. (See *Beyond the Relaxation Response* [New York: Berkley Books, 1985].)

So a person whose personal faith is based on the Bible might meditate this way:

Sometime in the morning, sit in a comfortable chair with your eyes closed, and concentrate on breathing regularly. As you breathe out, repeat silently a short word or phrase that conforms to your beliefs. For example, you might choose "The Lord is my shepherd" from the Twenty-third Psalm.

Continue repeating these words silently for ten to twenty minutes. If outside or distracting thoughts interfere with your focus on your belief words, don't become tense or upset. Maintain a passive attitude; gently turn away from the distraction and back to the biblical words you have chosen.

Then, engage in a second, similar session at some point later in the day.

This technique has produced dramatic results, according to presentations by Benson and others at a 1995 conference in Boston on the healing power of prayer. In addition to the previously mentioned physiologic changes (i.e., lower heart rate and blood pressure), more recent research has shown that eliciting the relaxation response has reduced visits to health maintenance organizations by 36 percent. Also, according to reports at the Boston conference, almost 40 percent of couples who believed they were infertile conceived within six months of practicing the technique. (See Associated Press release, December 6, 1995, published in *The Miami Herald*.)

Note: I know some Christians are uncomfortable with the concept of meditation because they associate it with transcendental meditation and other Eastern religious practices. But I believe it's important not to toss out a legitimate devotional practice just because another tradition uses something similar.

As I've reflected on the physiologic results of this type of meditation, I've often wondered if the approach being tested today at Harvard and elsewhere may not be similar to what King David used three thousand years ago. Throughout the Psalms, he strongly advocated meditating on God's "precepts," "statutes," "wonderful works," "name," "testimonies," and "word." (See Ps. 119:15, 23, 27, 55, 99, 148.) To me, David's approach seems distinct from ordinary prayers of confession or supplication—and closer to the meditative idea featured in current medical research of turning a short passage of Scripture over and over in your mind.

• Variations on simple meditation

Medical studies have been done on the effect of an advanced form of meditation known as "mindfulness meditation." This approach involves first establishing a breathing rhythm, as with simple meditation. Then, you repeat silently a personal belief word or phrase, such as "God is love." But instead of sticking to a mental repetition of this belief word, you allow your mind to move about among different ideas and feelings.

Usually, these thoughts are related in some way to the basic belief word. For example, if you begin with "God is love," your mind might move to a contemplation of the meaning of love—as described in 1 Corinthians 13—or the different manifestations of God in the Old and New Testaments.

In a review article produced by the MRC Applied Psychology Unit, Cambridge, England, the authors found encouraging evidence that mindfulness meditation can reduce stress and relieve depression. (See *Behavioral Research Therapy*, January 1995, pp. 25–39.)

Also, in a study conducted through the Department of Psychiatry, University of Massachusetts Medical Center, Worcester, twenty-two patients with anxiety disorders were put through an eight-week outpatient stress-reduction program, which was based on mindfulness meditation techniques. The subjects, who were followed up over a three-year period, showed significant improvements in their symptoms of anxiety and panic. The researchers concluded that a limited group stress-reduction program, based on mindfulness meditation, can have long-term beneficial effects in persons diagnosed with anxiety disorders. (See *General Hospital Psychiatry*, May 1995, pp. 192–200.)

• Comfortable rituals and peaceful contemplation

Sometimes, just finding a quiet, comfortable place to relax and contemplate is enough to reduce your stress levels. For example, people who have attended the traditional Japanese tea ceremonies report that the slow, ritualistic preparation and service of the tea have a calming effect on both observers and participants. The main purpose of the ceremony is to transform the tension-filled turmoil of daily life into a few moments of beauty and tranquillity.

Of course, many Westerners become restless in such an environment, especially if they fail to understand the purposes of the ritual. But those who can really get into the ceremony often feel their stresses slipping away. (See *Holistic Nursing Practice,* January 1996, pp. 30–7.)

I'm not as drawn to Japanese tea ceremonies as I am to other forms of contemplation, especially the contemplation of nature. When we are on vacation at our home in Beaver Creek, Colorado, I like to sit on the back deck and look out over the mountains, trees, and sky. Often, with my Bible on my lap, I'll turn to one of the nature psalms, such as Psalm 8, and contemplate the wonders of creation.

Even when I'm at my office in Dallas, I'll follow a similar practice every morning by closing my door, pulling out my Bible, and thinking and praying as I look out at the trees and ponds on our grounds at the Aerobics Center. Frequently, I'll find myself considering some of the deep paradoxes of Scripture, such as:

• Lose your life in order to save it.
• The leader must be the servant.
• The greatest will be the least.
• God's power is made perfect in our weakness.

Assuming this paradoxical mind-set (which, you'll recall from Chapter 3, is Step #1 in the Paradox Prescription) helps move me into a calm, meditative frame of mind. In the process, I know that the relaxation response lowers my heart rate and blood pressure.

At times as I'm following this practice, I might prefer to be in the solitude of Beaver Creek rather than the hullabaloo of Dallas. But whatever the setting, this quiet, regular contemplation provides me with a calming ritual, which helps me turn the bad stress in my life into a more positive and motivating force.

These first two approaches to using the mind to manage stress—cognitive-behavioral therapy and relaxation training—are the most commonly used techniques in medical research. They are likely to be powerful aids in dealing with your own bad stress.

But other stress-reduction strategies, which are often related to these first two categories, work quite well. Here is a sampling of additional "mental" ways of managing bad stress.

Reminiscence

Reflecting on positive experiences that you have had in the past can be effective in overcoming anxiety and other negative emotions produced by a stressful situation. This form of stress management, which may be done in a clinical setting in the form of "reminiscence sessions," may involve replaying in your mind pleasant encounters and events with family members or friends, successes at work, or good things that have been done for you and for which you are thankful.

In a case study reported in *Intensive Critical Care Nursing* (December 1995, pp. 341–3), a patient named Stuart had been in a hospital intensive care unit (ICU) for four weeks. The medical staff, which was finding it hard to wean him away from an artificial breathing device, reported that he was quite frightened, exhausted, and despondent. Depression, hopelessness, and apathy had overcome him.

Everything changed abruptly one day when the staff discovered a way to help Stuart escape temporarily from his situation: He began to engage in reminiscence sessions with the staff. Thinking back over the good experiences of his life and discussing them with the staff produced an almost immediate improvement. Three days later, he was breathing spontaneously and was prepared for discharge from the ICU.

Writing and Talking

Some of my patients rely heavily on daily journal writing as part of their devotionals and also as a means to objectify and analyze stress and other problems. The most accomplished practitioners of this art don't labor over their words as they write. Rather, they pour out their thoughts and feelings in an open and honest stream of consciousness without regard for punctuation, grammar, or form. Remember, if you use this approach, you should write for yourself (and perhaps God if you combine this technique with your devotions), not for a critique of your use of the English language.

Here's a variation on this approach for those who hate to write: Just talking about your stress-producing concern or problem—either to yourself or to a trusted friend—can fulfill a similar function.

Most psychiatric and mental health professionals use patient writing or talking in some form as a tool to encourage those suffering from bad stress to express their feelings and identify stressors. Also, narrative writing and journal writing (keeping a diary of feelings and emotions) can identify areas of conflict in one's life and clarify complicated issues. Writing can be used effectively with patients who are reluctant or embarrassed to speak openly in one-on-one interactions. (See *Journal of Psychosocial Nursing and Mental Health Services*, June 1996, pp. 31–5.)

In related studies by A. L. Mishara at the Department of Psychiatry, Case Western Reserve University, Cleveland, research has shown that writing about traumatic experiences can improve psychological and physiologic health. Mishara concluded that "healing through narration" and "opening up" on paper are practical means of transcending yourself and organizing your stressful experiences in new, healing ways. (See *American Journal of Psychotherapy*, Spring 1995, pp. 180–95.)

As for the talking cure, a concrete example of its success involved victims of the bombing of the World Trade Center in New York on February 26, 1993. At that time, hospitals were flooded with people who suffered from psychological as well as physical trauma. Nurses attending the victims talked with many about the traumatic incident, including the fear and angst they felt. The medical observers reported that this type of therapeutic talking became part of a cathartic process that helped the victims get better sooner and hasten healing of their unseen wounds. (See *Journal of Psychosocial Nursing and Mental Health Services*, June 1993, pp. 5–7.)

Music

On many occasions, I have encouraged patients who have problems with stress to turn off television or radio news, which can aggravate inner agitation and anxiety. Instead, I have suggested that they turn on soothing music at home, at the office during lunch, or in the car.

The car is a particularly good venue for this type of stress management if you are stuck frequently in traffic. As we saw in Chapter 2, a common stressor is commuting with its noise pollution, anger, and frustration.

This musical approach to stress finds strong support in the scientific literature. For example, in the *Journal of Post Anesthesia Nursing,* researchers noted that many patients in the surgical holding area become stressed out and anxious. But playing music there has been shown to reduce their anxiety.

In this 1994 study, one group of patients listened to music in the surgical holding area, while a second group did not. Those who filled their minds with music had significantly less stress and anxiety than did those who weren't exposed to the music. The researchers concluded that if music were available to all patients in this area, most would select the music option and would experience less anxiety. (See the December 1994 issue, pp. 340–3.)

Therapeutic Touch, Including Massage

From biblical times to the present, the practice of "laying on of hands" has often been linked to healing in a religious setting. In more recent years, modern medical experts confirm that touching patients in a compassionate, concerned way during regular medical treatment can hasten healing.

In a 1994 study of thirty-one patients at a Veterans Administration psychiatric facility in Maine, the participants were placed into therapeutic touch therapy, relaxation therapy, or a placebo group. After each of two fifteen-minute treatment sessions during a twenty-four-hour period, the subjects completed a self-reported anxiety evaluation and were rated for levels of muscle motor activity. (Excessive muscle movement can be an indicator of emotional agitation.)

The results: Therapeutic touch caused significant reductions in reported anxiety. Relaxation therapy also reduced self-reported anxiety and lowered the level of motor movement. The researchers concluded that both types of intervention are effective treatments for anxiety. (See *Archives of Psychiatric Nursing*, June 1994, pp. 184–9.)

In another study conducted at Healing Sciences Research International, Orinda, California, investigators measured the physiologic changes that occurred during therapeutic touch sessions. They found that physiologic activity, including hand and head temperatures and heart rate, showed a trend downward toward lower levels of arousal. (See *International Journal of Psychosomatics*, 1993, vol. 40, pp. 47–55.)

A related touching technique—massage—may reduce symptoms of stress. In a small-scale study of stress in a hospital labor ward, twenty-five staff members were asked about their stress at work. Eighty percent said they felt stressed out, mainly because of overwork. They said talking to others was their main way of coping, yet only half felt they were adequately supported at work.

Then, the participants were offered a twenty-minute massage, and all reported afterward that they felt it helped reduce their feelings of stress. The self-reporting was supported by measurements of their heart rate, which dropped by an average of twelve beats per minute during the massage sessions. (See *Modern Midwife*, February 1995, pp. 7–10.)

Massage may be combined effectively with other stress-reduction techniques. In a 1994 case study conducted by the Department of Psychology and Human Ecology, Cameron University, Lawton, Oklahoma, physicians treated a sixteen-year-old boy who suffered from five years of hair loss. His condition, known as alopecia areata, is generally considered a result of defects in the autoimmune process.

Three treatment techniques were used with the boy: hair massage, relaxation procedures, and monetary rewards. His condition was evaluated after seven months without the treatments, and then after seven months with the treatments. The combined treatments reduced hair loss markedly after three months, and new hair growth occurred during the last four months. (See *Psychological Reports*, June 1994, pp. 1315–8.)

Group Support

There are many ways to use groups to lower individual anxiety, including formal therapy and informal support group experiences. In formal group therapy, a professional therapist may lead the participants through a process of confronting their fears, redefining them, and working together to help individuals in the group overcome stress.

In a less formal setting, the members of religious or other philosophically like-minded groups will typically meet regularly for open, highly personal discussions. Common ground rules include absolute confidentiality, honesty in sharing, and a willingness to be vulnerable with one another.

For example, some of my Christian patients are involved in prayer-and-share groups or koinonia groups. These small groups, which usually involve three to eight people, will first share their concerns—especially the stresses that develop from personal, work, or family challenges. Then, they will discuss and analyze the problems based on the group's understanding of the Bible and other religious sources. Finally, the group will pray about the concerns.

The support of others through these group channels can be decisive in lowering levels of stress. A 1994 study by the Department of Oral Epidemiology and Public Health, Royal Dental College, Aarhus University, Denmark, focused on group therapy treatments for dental anxiety. Thirty group therapy patients were compared with sixty-eight individual treatment patients and forty-five controls.

The researchers found that the group therapy patients experienced a greater reduction in dental anxiety than the individual treatment patients. But the dropout rate was much higher in group therapy. (See *Community Dental and Oral Epidemiology,* August 1994, pp. 258–62.)

Humor

The use of humor to overcome bad stress might be regarded as a form of cognitive-behavioral therapy in that humor can act as a distraction or substitute for worry. But I also like to highlight humor as a separate category because joking and laughing can be so important in turning a bad, "down" mood into an outlook that is at least acceptable.

For example, researchers at the National Pediatric and Family HIV Resource Center, University of Medicine and Dentistry, New Jersey Medical School, Newark, reported on nurses working with patients suffering from HIV disease. The nurses frequently felt under stress and frustrated, even though on the whole, they regarded their work as rewarding.

A review article on this situation, published in *Nursing Clinics in North America* (March 1996, pp. 243–51), revealed that humor—along with group support, individual stress-management strategies, and spirituality—helped the nurses maintain their energy and enthusiasm for their nursing practice.

Dealing with a related issue, researchers at the Department of Anthropology, Drew University, Madison, New Jersey, studied the effect of the Big Apple Circus Clown Care Unit on children who were patients in New York City hospitals. The "clown doctors" used strange and colorful costumes, music, sleight of hand, puppet helpers, and ventriloquism.

The researchers, who drew comparisons with non-Western healers and shamans, found that using "clown doctors" may enhance the effects of medical treatment, especially for children. (See *Medical Anthropology Quarterly*, December 1995, pp. 462–75.)

Fostering an Attitude of Expectancy and Hope

A positive attitude and sense of positive expectation should always underlie every treatment for stress, whether it involves psychological techniques or "hard" medical interventions, such as drug therapy. The greater the sense of hope in the patient, the greater the likelihood of a successful and faster cure.

In a 1994 study published in *Social Sciences and Medicine* (July 1995, pp. 249–60), California researchers looked into the impact of the expectations of patients and a "spiritual healer" on mental and physical health. The results of the three-week study suggested that a high sense of positive expectancy by both the patient and the healer was an important predictor and factor in the healing process. In this study, 75 percent of the conditions reported were organic disorders, which usually would not disappear within the time limits set for the study.

• • • •

As you can see from our discussion up to this point, no clear line in the medical literature separates mental and spiritual techniques for lowering stress and healing disease. In fact, many of the nonspiritual approaches we have discussed—

such as meditation, contemplation, group sharing, and a sense of hope—are also deeply rooted in Judeo-Christian history and tradition, and could fit easily into a strictly religious setting.

Of course, this conclusion shouldn't be surprising if one makes the traditional Christian and Hebrew assumption that God is God of the whole person—whether the mind, the emotions, the body, or the human spirit. Healing accounts throughout the Old and New Testaments often weave the practical and medicinal with the spiritual. The healing of King Hezekiah through prayer and a poultice of figs is a case in point. (See 2 Kings 20:1–7.)

Sometimes, as modern medical researchers try to sort out the spiritual dimensions of healing, their attempts can lead to interesting findings that have particular relevance to our search for antidotes to stress. So let's join these scientists as they try to find the spiritual spark in healing stress-related complaints.

Finding the Spiritual Spark

Is there medical evidence that prayer and other specifically religious practices can really help to heal the ravages of stress?

Increasingly, scientists are answering yes to this question. Their latest revelations about spirituality and stress emphasize the importance of these three components of religious experience: (1) personal faith; (2) religious ritual and practice; and (3) prayer.

Personal Faith

A number of studies have shown that a deeply held personal faith in God can reduce stress. A medical news article in the *Journal of the American Medical Association* (May 24–31, 1995, pp. 1561–62) reported on a study by Dr. Harold G. Koenig of Duke University Medical Center, Durham, North Carolina, who had investigated religious coping among disabled adults over age sixty-five. He defined religious coping as the use of religious practice and experience—such as prayer, faith in God, and Bible reading—to combat bad stress.

Koenig found that disabled older people were less likely to become depressed if they scored high in religious coping. Also, he noted that those who made ongoing use of religious coping techniques became less depressed over time.

Another physician featured in this report, Dr. Jeffrey S. Levin of Eastern Virginia Medical School, Norfolk, reviewed medical research on the effect of religious faith on the outcomes of such conditions as heart disease, cancer, tuberculosis, and suicide. He reported that of twenty-seven studies in which patients had some religious connection, twenty-two showed a significant positive effect on disease. As a result, he concluded that a "lack of religious involvement seems to be a risk factor [for poorer health]" (p. 1562).

Further scientific support for the power of faith can be found in a 1995 report in *Psychosomatic Medicine.* This study revealed that 232 elderly patients, who had been through open-heart surgery and had strong religious beliefs, had a survival rate three times higher than people without a faith. (See *The New York Times,* February 4, 1995, p. 9.)

A stress connection was apparent in the study because of the twenty-one patients who died in the six months following surgery, most experienced cardiac arrhythmias, or irregularities in the heartbeat.

The psychiatrist who headed the study, Dr. Thomas Oxman of Dartmouth Medical School, Hanover, New Hampshire, concluded, "It may be that having faith translates into your being more soothed psychologically. If your mind is calmer, that might make arrhythmias less likely."

From such studies, it has become apparent that a deeply felt, "intrinsic" or inner faith can be a positive factor in health, including stress management. But researchers are still trying to describe the precise features of such a strong faith. Merely attending church or claiming to be a strong believer is usually not enough (though some exceptions to this point are indicated in the following section). On the other hand, a faith that produces a strong sense of optimism or hope can make a difference in physical and emotional health.

These observations are only the beginning of the story. Obviously, further research will be necessary if we hope to make any real progress toward resolving the fascinating question that medical researchers continue to ask: What kind of faith produces the best health?

Religious Ritual and Practice

There is no question that a strong inner faith usually seems more healthful and a better antidote for stress than mere outward observance. However, some people, including certain ethnic groups, appear to respond well to membership in a specific church, to certain rituals, or even to regular church attendance.

In a report in the *Journal of the National Medical Association* (November 1994, pp. 825–31), researchers from Wayne State University found that among African-American males, three types of religious involvement could be beneficial to health: (1) denominational affiliation, (2) frequency of church attendance, and (3) overall religiosity.

The results of the study showed fewer symptoms of depression among those with a denominational affiliation. Those who never or rarely attended church were more likely to engage in unhealthful habits, such as smoking or drinking alcohol daily.

Religious rituals can provide a particularly supportive cushion for people who move from one culture to another—while removing a ritual can lead to serious health problems. A refugee woman who moved from Ethiopia to Israel underwent numerous traumatic emotional upheavals, including losing her baby and being prevented from undergoing traditional purification rituals in her new land. As a result, she suffered signs and symptoms of post-traumatic stress disorder, including respiratory problems and depression.

Her treatment included receiving psychotherapy and being allowed to undergo her purification rituals. Within thirty months, her stress problems had dissipated, and she had stabilized emotionally. (See the *British Journal of Medicine and Psychology*, June 1995, pp. 135–42.)

Prayer

Perhaps the most intriguing component of the kind of faith that can produce healing—including the effective treatment of stress—is prayer. Consequently, scientists are intensifying their efforts to see whether the effects of prayer can be measured or quantified.

For example, researchers have launched studies at the University of Arkansas to see if human muscle cells will respond to prayer at a distance. Also, through the support of the National Institutes of Health, scientists at the University of New Mexico are examining the effects of the prayers of Catholics, Protestants, and Jews on alcoholics and drug users. In addition, investigators at Temple University are studying whether prayer helps infants at risk from serious neonatal conditions. (See *The Wall Street Journal,* December 20, 1995, p. B1.)

Some completed studies have already suggested that health benefits may be connected with prayer. One of the best known in medical circles involved research in the mid-1980s by the cardiologist Randolph Byrd. He arranged for evangelical Christians to pray for nearly four hundred heart patients in San Francisco. Then, they were compared with a control group that did not receive prayer.

Dr. Byrd reported in the *Southern Medical Journal* that the group that had been the subject of the prayers needed fewer antibiotics and had less risk of accumulating fluid in the lungs than the group that was not prayed for. Also, no one who received prayer needed artificial breathing machines, while twelve of those in the control group did. (See *The Wall Street Journal* report, p. B2.)

More recent studies have confirmed that some sort of scientifically measurable healing may occur with prayer. For example, in a 1994 investigation at the Pain Clinic, Helsinki University Central Hospital, Finland, twenty-four patients with chronic pain of unknown origin ("idiopathic" pain) were divided into two groups; one received spiritual healing therapy, and the other received no active treatment.

At the end of the study the researchers found a minor decrease in the intake of drugs and an improvement in sleep patterns among patients for whom the healer prayed. Also, the prayed-for patients experienced a decrease in their feelings of hopelessness.

The researchers concluded that the spiritual healing efforts certainly caused no harm and were helpful in relieving subjective stress-related feelings and symptoms among the patients with chronic pain. (See *Clinical Journal of Pain,* December 1994, pp. 296–302.)

According to a 1994 report in the *International Journal of Psychosomatics* (vol. 41, pp. 68–75), California researchers from Healing Sciences Research International found that prayers uttered at a distance were associated with a number of physiologic changes in twenty-one subjects. The participants, who were blind to the true nature of the experiment, experienced a slight decrease in stress-responsive measurements, including blood volume pulse, a lower heart rate, and electromagnetic energy in four muscle regions.

Of course, there are limits to how far we can go in proving the efficacy of prayer or other spiritual health strategies, either for people with stress-related illnesses or for people with any other complaints. But this limitation will hardly worry persons with deep faith. Those with strong religious beliefs don't need scientists to gather evidence that prayer works. They know from personal experience that prayer and other spiritual disciplines are effective.

In any event, when the various mental and spiritual possibilities for managing stress are taken together, they present a formidable arsenal of weapons against stress. To see further how these and other techniques can overcome stress in your life, let's turn to the next step in your Paradox Prescription—Step #6—which involves becoming an expert in employing "depressurizing tactics" in daily high-stress situations, including the work environment.

CHAPTER 7

RELEASE AND RETREAT: THE TWO GREAT SECRETS OF HIGHLY PRODUCTIVE PEOPLE

The power exerted by the Paradox Prescription reaches full force with job-related stress. Two great paradoxes provide the key to inner tranquillity and balance in the world of work:

First, if you *release* your ambitions, you will reach them more easily.

Second, if you *retreat* from your work, you will become more productive.

Although we'll consider many stressors and treatments for job stress throughout this chapter, these two central paradoxes underlie all else. Don't be concerned at this point if you don't quite grasp their full meaning or how they might work in your life. First, we have to explore what job stress is and where it comes from. Then you will be in a position to understand the true meanings of *release* and *retreat*—and how these principles may work in your life.

The best way I know to introduce what a burden job stress can place on our shoulders and how stress may be overcome is to share a few of my experiences. I have said that I sometimes feel I have become a kind of black belt in fighting the stress in my life. The following "autobiography of stress" will give you an idea of how I have earned this rank.

An Autobiography of Stress

My life story could be written by moving from one stressful incident to the next. Being a type A personality, who is driven by overachievement, overwork, and perfectionism, I have become a magnet for bad stress.

To be sure, I sympathize with whatever stressful situations you are currently confronting. Furthermore, I know that any heavy personal pressure can pose a serious threat to emotional and physical well-being. But at the same time, I have to say to you, "I've been there."

On a number of occasions, I've teetered on the very edge of career failure, rejection by professional peers, and even bankruptcy. I could, quite literally, fill an entire book with tales of my battles with the dragons of pressure, strain, and tension. However, this thumbnail autobiography will feature only three of my most significant stressful encounters:

- My fight with the air force to get my first book, *Aerobics,* published and recognized, including a spat along the way with TV host Barbara Walters;
- my battle against opposition by the medical establishment as I attempted to establish preventive medicine, including treadmill testing, as a legitimate area of practice;
- the chilling specter of imminent bankruptcy.

I've worried, lost sleep, and at times despaired of hope. But somehow, despite the relentless onslaught of a multitude of heavyweight stressors, I believe I have emerged a stronger and perhaps even a wiser person. Here's how it happened.

The Battle of the Book

Back in the mid-1960s, when I was a career officer and flight surgeon in the U.S. Air Force, I began to conduct research in Texas on the exercise needs of our pilots and astronauts. After evaluating thousands of military personnel at every level of physical fitness, I came up with the aerobics point system for improving cardiovascular fitness. The emphasis was on a graduated program of conditioning through endurance activities, including jogging, running, and cycling.

The results were staggering. By 1968, there were 27,000 military people in the program, and their physical conditions were improving by leaps and bounds. About that time, word about my work leaked to the secular news media and publishers, and my phone started ringing off the hook. That was when my career star began to rise—and also when the trouble started.

A booklet describing the aerobics program had already been published and circulated by the air force, but I felt it was also important to communicate the principles I had discovered to the public at large. That meant doing a book for an outside publisher, and M. Evans and Company of New York made me an offer I felt I couldn't refuse.

By the time the hardback edition of the book was published, my life had changed forever. My then editor, now agent, Herbert M. Katz, had sold rights to *Reader's Digest,* Book of the Month Club, and Bantam paperbacks. If I thought life as an air force major and doctor had involved pressure before, I had a big surprise coming.

First of all, the powers that be in the air force resisted publication of the book. I didn't quite understand their rationale, but everywhere I turned, I met a roadblock. You can never fathom the full meaning of red tape until you try to use military channels to do something a little unusual.

Whatever the reason for the opposition, I finally managed to get grudging permission to go ahead with the book, primarily because I had the support of the former surgeon general of the air force, Lt. Gen. Richard L. Bohannon. As a matter of fact, Lieutenant General Bohannon wrote the introduction to the book, which came out in 1968 under the title *Aerobics.*

But my troubles with the air force weren't over yet. Representatives of the news industry showed considerable interest in interviewing me about the book, and one of the first electronic newspeople I encountered was Barbara Walters. I was looking forward to the interview, which was scheduled for the radio, but from the moment I sat down in front of the microphone, I knew something was wrong.

Although she questioned me in a straightforward way about the aerobics program, I sensed she was rather hostile. She never looked me in the eye, and her questions were considerably more skeptical than I felt the program warranted.

When we went off the air, I asked, "What's wrong? I don't understand your response to my program."

"I know all about you," she said. "You're a fake. We know the air force has no interest in your program because we called the surgeon general's office, and they said they don't support you. They said it's just Cooper doing it for his own gain."

I pulled out the official air force manual that contained my program and tossed it over to her. "Does that look like they don't support it?" I asked.

She took some time to look over the manual—throwing in an approving comment, "Interesting . . . interesting," every now and then. She got up and left the room for a few minutes. When she returned, she asked, "Can you be on the *Today* show next Thursday?"

I ended up on *Today* for an interview lasting about ten minutes with Barbara Walters and Hugh Downs. When I returned to the Bantam offices, I learned there had been ten thousand new requests for the book as a result of my appearance on the show. That kicked off the first book and soon helped place the book on the national best-seller lists.

Obviously, there was a happy ending to this publishing saga, but believe me, I felt plenty of bad stress along the way. I was constantly caught in the grip of situations that I couldn't control. The decisions to approve publication of the book and to schedule me for major national media appearances were largely out of my hands.

How did I manage this stress? As a relatively young air force major, I wasn't as experienced at dealing with such situations as I am now. But I took my first steps toward learning to release events and decisions that I couldn't control, no matter how important I perceived them to be to my future. If you try to control issues that are out of your control, you've set an impossible task for yourself, and you can be sure that your bad stress will build to unbearable levels.

This kind of release involves a two-step process: (1) deciding to let go of what you can't control, and (2) "dropping" the issue or stressor into "hands" other than your own.

First, in order to let go, you have to identify precisely what it is that you can't control. In my case, I knew that the ultimate air force decision was out of my hands. Also, I knew I couldn't force Barbara Walters to put me on the *Today* show.

Identifying the out-of-control issues was fairly easy. Then I said to myself, "I'm letting you go."

Second, I had to figure out where I was going to "drop" the stressors that were beyond my control, and that was the hard part. You see, if you just let a problem or worry go without pushing it in a particular, productive direction, the chances are, it will boomerang right back to you.

In what direction did I release my stressors? I chose an earthly direction and a heavenly one. I let my friend, Lieutenant General Bohannon, know about my problems, and I asked for his help. In effect, I released my problems with the air force to him. And I released *all* my concerns to God in prayer. Ultimately, I believed even then, in that early stage of my spiritual development, that while many things are out of my control, nothing is out of His control. Of course, I didn't know what His will was in the book publishing and promotion matters. But I knew if I could effectively cast all my cares on Him—and reorder my priorities so that my need to succeed with a book came second to my submission to God's will—I would find a powerful antidote to my stress. (See 1 Peter 5:7.)

Finally, as I've suggested several times before, I don't believe it helps—and it usually hurts—to try to fight uncontrollable forces head-on. You must think and act more paradoxically by backing off instead of locking horns with some issues. Yet at the same time, you must stay active and assume a jujitsulike fighting mentality against your bad stress, one in which you identify and let go of the things you can't control while you nudge the stressors in a productive direction.

This may mean putting a trusted confidant or expert in charge, as I did with Lieutenant General Bohannon. Or it may mean finding a spiritual "home" for your concern. You may feel comfortable just saying fatalistically, "Whatever will be will be." Or you may choose a more traditional, religious approach as I did.

These, then, are some basic ways to "release" a stressor. But there are many variations—as you'll see in the next part of my "autobiography."

The Opposition of the Medical Establishment

Soon after the publication of *Aerobics,* I realized that my destiny was not going to be with the air force. I wanted to do so many things in preventive medicine, and I couldn't pursue a lot of them in the military.

So I left the air force and moved to Dallas in 1970—taking with me the treadmill I had been using to test pilots and astronauts. On its face, the move was crazy. I was turning my back on thirteen years in the military and the certainty of an eventual pension. Despite my problems in getting my book published, I was on the verge of being promoted to full colonel. And there I was, tossing aside those prospects and heading for a new city with a pregnant wife, no insurance, a five-year-old daughter, and a dog.

But I had a dream that I wanted to follow. I set up shop in a little two-room office in North Dallas on December 6, 1970, and I began doing stress tests with my treadmill. The patients were few and far between at first, but before long, that changed. The exercise electrocardiogram (ECG) I obtained from each stress test enabled me to find a few hidden heart problems and save a few lives. As the word about my practice spread, my patient caseload started to increase.

A little success may attract some attention, but in my case, the attention was not the kind I wanted. Almost immediately, I got flak from some Dallas doctors, especially cardiologists, who apparently felt I was encroaching on their territory.

Among other things, they argued that I was not a board-certified cardiologist and I was unqualified to perform the stress tests. They charged that because I was having my patients walk to exhaustion on the treadmills, I was actually endangering their lives.

To understand why the controversy grew so heated, you need to know a little history of the issue. The concept of exercising to exhaustion to get a more accurate ECG was quite new at the time. Most doctors felt that anyone employing stress electrocardiography should only use the Masters Two Step test and then not allow patients to exceed 85 percent of their "predicted maximal heart rate" (PMHR). This rate can be calculated by using the formula PMHR equals 220 minus the patient's age. In other words, only submaximal stress testing was acceptable among the majority of physicians I encountered in those days. In contrast, I was advocating maximal performance treadmill stress testing.

The dispute became so intense that my opponents tried to force me to stop stress testing by requiring me to go before the Dallas County Medical Board of Censors. There was even a possibility that if the Board had ruled against me, I might have lost some of my medical privileges and been required to change my practice of preventive medicine.

As I expected, the charges were dropped for lack of evidence, but that didn't stop the opposition from going after me. The military had been bad enough, but the doctors were trying to run me out of town! One was passing around rumors that I wasn't a physician at all, but rather was a Ph.D. Another said I had been dishonorably discharged from the air force.

Needless to say, the attacks placed extreme stress on me. I knew that the doctors felt threatened by my presence because some of the patients I was seeing had originally been theirs. In reality, the whole episode was probably the result of professional jealousy.

As though it were yesterday, I still recall how emotionally and spiritually disturbed I became. To begin with, I was working too long—twelve to fourteen hours per day. Because my work had become my life, everything else got out of balance. My priorities went like this: Work was first, family was a distant second, and God was completely out of the picture. I was praying very little during that period, and when I did pray, it was on the run, usually a "foxhole prayer" to ask for help out of a crisis.

The only thing that stabilized me was my regular running. I ran five or six days for a total of twelve to fifteen miles per week. The exercise, and the exercise alone, enabled me to burn up my stress hormones and get sufficient sleep at night. I really believe that if I hadn't been running during that period, my health would have broken under the pressure.

The attacks on me faded as my fellow doctors began to see the virtues of treadmill stress testing. The medical climate in the mid-1970s was changing toward a greater acceptance of and interest in preventive medicine. Over time, I saw the hostility of a number of physicians turn into grudging respect, and even a source of referrals for my practice.

I give my commitment to aerobic exercise great credit for helping me make it through the early trials and tribulations of civilian medical practice. In a sense, I guess you could say I retreated from my job stress daily by turning away from work and toward exercise. The regular shifting of mental and emotional gears was decisive in helping me keep my stress at manageable levels during the crisis.

But exercise wasn't nearly enough to carry me through another crisis that hit in the late 1980s—a crisis that very nearly brought financial ruin, even though by this time my operation had grown considerably with a large staff of doctors and other personnel.

The Brink of Bankruptcy

After we established the Cooper Clinic, Cooper Aerobics Center, and Cooper Institute for Aerobics Research at our current location on Preston Road in North Dallas, our business really began to boom. We were treating thousands of patients, had three thousand members in our Aerobics Center fitness club, and were grossing several million dollars a year in revenues.

But then, disaster struck. I received a phone call at 4:00 A.M. on New Year's Day in 1981: "Dr. Cooper, the Aerobics Center is on fire!"

The blaze started in the laundry room, but fortunately, the damage was limited to one part of the Center. Still, we had to suspend operations while repairs were made, and our insurance company pegged the loss at $1.4 million.

Just after the fire, someone from a local radio station called me, and I pledged over the air, "This won't destroy us. We'll build the Center back bigger and better than ever."

Those self-assured, prideful words came back to haunt me. We did indeed build it back to three times its former size, and our membership in the club rose to 3,600 members, with a two-year waiting list and a staff of hundreds. We accomplished all that just as the recession hit in the mid- to late 1980s, and we felt the downturn as much as other companies. Many of our members were corporate sponsored, and they either lost this fringe benefit or lost their jobs. So our membership declined, and our patient load went down as well.

In that period, banks and thrifts were falling like flies around the country. Even though we were feeling some pressure, I wasn't particularly worried. We had spent more than $6 million for a guest lodge on our property and were still generating adequate revenue. I hadn't missed a payment on my business debts, which at that point stood at nearly $10 million.

Before I knew it, a larger, out-of-state bank purchased my lender, and the new people started going over their outstanding loans with a microscope. In 1988, representatives of the bank contacted me and said, "Dr. Cooper, we have done an evaluation of your operation, and we don't like what we see."

"I haven't missed a payment," I said. "What's wrong? I'm not in arrears, so why are you getting on my back?"

"This is a different ball game with different players," they said.

What they really meant was that they didn't like the idea that I had secured my loan at a very low interest rate, and they were unhappy with the money they were making. It was clear that they wanted to call my note and put my money to work with someone else at a much higher rate of interest.

They started pressing me into a corner by giving me a list of changes I had to make to keep the loan intact. I was supposed to upgrade our facilities in various ways, such as putting in more computers and hiring additional help.

Rather than argue, I met their demands. Even though it cost me a total of $600,000, I conformed to the letter to the changes they wanted.

In January 1989, I asked, "How does my situation look?"

"You're doing great," they said.

But in April 1989, they dropped a bomb. They told me my loan had been assigned to still another bank, and the new bank was ready to call the loan. In short, they said, I should prepare for bankruptcy.

I had to spend *another* $600,000 over the next three years to prepare for possible bankruptcy. That involved liquidating all my savings and preparing absolutely precise financial statements. I was told that if I erred by more than $10,000 on those statements, the government could accuse me of falsifying documents and put me in jail. Talk about pressure!

Those three years were literally hell on earth for me. My personal net worth went from several million to zero. The new bank turned up the pressure. They notified me formally that my note was to be called, and they declared they were going to foreclose on the Aerobics Center property and put a lock on the gate.

I was terrified, even though my bankruptcy attorney said, "They can't do that. You have at least thirty days to respond."

I didn't know whether to believe him or not. In any case, I didn't sleep for two straight nights after that first foreclosure notice.

That marked the beginning of a dark three-year night for me. I could see no light at the end of any tunnel. No one stepped forward to help me financially. The only recourse I had was to fall back completely on God. Millie and I prayed more during that period than we had in the preceding twenty years.

Eventually, I realized that the most important step I had to take was not financial, but spiritual. I prayed, "Lord, you gave me all this property as a custodian. It's yours. I am only handling it for you. If I lose it, that's just your way of taking it back."

In other words, I *released* that property into God's hands. I had to relinquish any pride of ownership I had, any moral right over my material things. From that moment, I felt free of the need to possess the business and medical practice that I had built. At least I knew I still had a profession and wouldn't be on the welfare rolls.

A few weeks later, the bank sent me a second foreclosure notice. I didn't sleep for one whole night after that one. A third notice came along shortly afterward, and it bothered me, but I managed to get to sleep all right.

When the fourth notice arrived, I ignored it. I could see that they were harassing me in the hope that I would make a wrong move. The best strategy was obviously to release the matter to the hands of my attorney.

He told me not to meet with anyone from the bank or even talk with its representatives. "Let us take the brunt of this," he said. "They will call you names and try to make you angry and say something you'll regret later."

In the meantime, on the advice of counsel, I stopped making payments on my note directly to the bank, though I put the money into an escrow account with the bank. That way, the bankers couldn't touch it, but they could see I wasn't spending it. The money would be there for them if we could reach an equitable settlement.

As the negotiations proceeded, my attorney kept a list of possible lawsuits I could bring against the bank. They made so many mistakes in dealing with me that we had several good causes of action by the time the bank finally indicated a willingness to settle. One term of the final agreement was that I wouldn't file suit against the bank!

All these financial crises are well behind me. The debts have been refinanced, and the Aerobics Center and our other operations are on a sound footing. Furthermore, I must say that, despite the pain and bad stress I experienced, in some ways I'm thankful for being put through that nerve-racking challenge. Now that it's over, I sense that my priorities are much more in order. Given my Christian worldview, I know that I can handle heavy stress like this bankruptcy threat well only through the resources afforded by my faith.

But this is just my story. You have to look deep inside yourself and explore your philosophy of life to find your way to overcoming the most serious job-related stressors. Sometimes, you may go to the brink of disaster and somehow come back, as I did with the Aerobics Center. Other times, you may end up losing the career achievement you hold most dear. Whatever the result, the twin paradoxical themes of release and retreat are always available to usher you through the darkest hour.

Now, let's move from my situation to yours. Many times, stress on the job doesn't appear quite as dramatically as I have depicted in my "autobiography." Rather than face a total loss of your business or career, you may confront a slow, steady deterioration of enthusiasm, motivation, and satisfaction with your work—or what is known in the research literature as "burnout." What does this involve, and how can you deal with it?

What Is Burnout—and Why Is It So Bad?

Burnout on the job is often described as a syndrome characterized by emotional exhaustion, a sense of depersonalization, and feelings of reduced personal accomplishment. One 1994 study of general dental practitioners in southeast England, for instance, identified these signs in many of the more than three hundred participants in the investigation. (See *British Dental Journal,* November 19, 1994, pp. 372–7.)

Other possible symptoms of burnout include physical fatigue, gastrointestinal problems, and various aches and pains associated with other types of stress. A study at the Cardiovascular and Hypertension Center, New York Hospital-Cornell University Medical College, New York, established that job strain can raise systolic blood pressure. (See *Scandinavian Journal of Work Environment Health,* October 1994, pp. 349–63.)

After evaluating 262 full-time male employees in eight work sites, the researchers found that the employees experiencing job strain had systolic blood pressures that were 6.7 mm Hg higher than other employees. (The systolic reading is the "top" or first blood pressure measurement. So if your pressure is 135/75, the systolic reading is 135, while the diastolic reading is 75.)

The work stressors may even become so heavy that more serious emotional disorders result. A case in point: A 1996 news report out of Great Britain revealed that John Walker, a fifty-nine-year-old social worker, had been awarded $270,000 after suffering a work-related nervous breakdown that forced him to quit his job. The court ruled that his employer was liable for levying "impossible workloads," which increased stress. (See *The Wall Street Journal,* November 19, 1996, p. 1.)

So burnout can definitely damage your emotional and physical health and well-being. But what signals should you look for to know that burnout may be on the way? It's best not to wait for any of the symptoms I've mentioned to occur before you act. The best preventive approach is to know your stress "danger zones" at work and try to avoid or correct them as soon as possible.

Know Your Stress Danger Zones

Rather than focus on what *might* be danger zones for bad stress at work, let me stick to the hard evidence and mention some of the *known* problem areas. These have all appeared in recent years in studies that have delved into the causes of burnout. Then, using them as your starting point, you can branch out to analyze your work environment and compile your personal list of potential job stressors.

Job Uncertainty and Job Loss

Among the patients I see on a daily basis at the Cooper Clinic, fear and anxiety about the security of their jobs combine to be a major source of stress. If a person has lost his job, I can quite literally see it in his eyes and face, and in the way he looks and walks. Loss of appetite and loss of sleep undoubtedly contribute to the stressed-out look.

My patients aren't alone in these fears. According to the Bureau of Labor Statistics, in the most recently studied three-year period 4.5 million workers who had been with their employers at least three years were displaced. In other words, their jobs were eliminated. Also, according to this study, during their first year of unemployment, only one-third of the workers found another job that paid as much or more than the one they lost.

Another problem is that as workers age, many are being "encouraged" or forced to retire early, well before the traditional age of sixty-five. Those who have to quit their jobs before they are ready often develop symptoms of stress, and the loss of meaning or of constructive occupation may drive them to an early grave.

I recall vividly many of the enlisted air force retirees I counseled while I was on active duty. They were often only thirty-eight to forty years of age when they left the service, but they became so depressed at the prospect of starting over that they started looking like old men.

A similar theme is being played out in the civilian world. According to a 1991 report from the Employee Benefit Research Institute, almost 40 percent of all workers are finished with their chosen career jobs by age fifty-five. Further, almost 60 percent had left their career jobs by age sixty. As a result, many of these people face lower incomes and more economic uncertainty—which can be serious sources of stress.

Because of such trends, former Labor Secretary Robert Reich has called America's middle class "the anxious class, most of whom hold jobs, but who are justifiably uneasy about their own standing and fearful for their children's futures." (See *Tropic* magazine, October 15, 1995.)

Shift Work

Working on rotating shifts, in which sleep rhythms are disrupted, may be a risk factor for heart attacks among women, according to a report in the December 1, 1995, issue of *Circulation,* the journal of the American Heart Association.

This Harvard Medical School investigation evaluated approximately 79,000 female nurses, aged thirty to fifty-five, 59 percent of whom had worked irregular shifts for more than six years. The researchers found that the participants on shift work were up to 70 percent more likely to have heart attacks than their colleagues who didn't have this type of job. According to the scientists, disrupting the body's biological clock acts as a stressor by causing excess production of stress hormones.

In my clinical practice I have observed that both male and female patients who work irregular hours, with constantly changing sleep and meal schedules, are more vulnerable to stress. In other words, regardless of gender, shift workers are likely to have more symptoms such as headaches, backaches, and fatigue—and may very well be placing themselves at risk of serious disease.

Time and Deadline Pressure

If the hours you work are excessively long, or if you are constantly under deadline pressure, you are more likely to experience signs of bad stress.

For example, in a 1994 study conducted at Wright State University School of Medicine, Dayton, Ohio, researchers looked into how burnout may contribute to the impairment of the effectiveness of physicians, as well as patient dissatisfaction. After giving a test on burnout to fifty residency-trained family physicians, the investigators concluded that time demands on doctors were an important factor in exhaustion and the impairment of their performances. (See *Family Practice and Research Journal,* September 1994, pp. 213–22.)

Workload

A problem directly related to time pressure involves the burdens accompanying a heavy workload. South African researchers found that speech-language therapists and audiologists with heavy caseloads—who *perceived* themselves to be under great work pressure—were the most susceptible to burnout. Emotional exhaustion was a primary symptom. (See *South African Journal of Communications Disorders,* 1993, vol. 40, pp. 71–84.)

A 1994 comparison of Canadian and Jordanian nurses came to similar conclusions. In *Health Care Women International* (September-October, pp. 413–21), the investigators reported that for both groups, the main factors determining burnout were excessive workloads, unsatisfying work, and uncertainties about career future.

Heavy workloads may combine with other factors to increase the risk of emotional exhaustion and eventual burnout. In another study of hospital workers (published in *ANNA Journal,* October 1994, pp. 325–36), the researchers concluded that the main factors contributing to emotional exhaustion were a low sense of coherence (sense of meaning or direction on the job), lack of staff support, personal stress levels, *and* a heavy workload.

Control Problems

Everyone operates better at work when he or she has a significant degree of control over work assignments. Also, those who have an unusually high need to control circumstances and outcomes involving their employees, their colleagues, and even their employers are at an even greater risk of stress problems when they lose control.

I'm reminded of one of my patients who had been extremely successful in building his own business, but in the process, he had fallen into the habit of micromanaging his employees. Instead of delegating tasks to them, he was always looking over their shoulders, monitoring their progress, and telling them what to do.

As a result, he was working eighteen-hour days: He had to get in early and leave late because during the main part of the day, he was always up to his eyeballs in his employees' problems.

The physical and emotional toll on him was overwhelming. He had quit exercising entirely because he refused to take time away from his business. He was sleeping poorly because he delayed going to bed when he arrived home at night. He felt he had to sit down in front of his TV with a cocktail for an hour or so before bedtime in order to "decompress." As you might expect, his family life was nonexistent. His children were always asleep when he arrived home, and his wife was asleep by the time he crawled into bed.

Fortunately, before he began to experience serious physical symptoms, the early signs of stress, especially excessive fatigue, drove him to see his doctor. During the interview after the physical exam, his account of his poor work habits raised a red flag with his physician. The doctor warned the patient that he was riding for a fall with his health if he continued on his present course.

The "prescription" the entrepreneur was given was purely preventive: He was instructed that it was *essential* for him to relinquish control over his business to his employees and to cut back significantly on his work hours and workload. His business was still growing quite rapidly, and if he failed to delegate, he would almost certainly face serious physical, emotional, and family problems in the near future.

Unlike many entrepreneurs in similar situations, this man listened to his doctor. Now he has cut back his workday to about eleven hours, and on some Saturdays and Sundays, he works only half a day! He still has a tendency to try to exercise too much control over others, but his energy levels and healthy sleep patterns have returned.

Giving up control is one of the most difficult steps for a hard-charging, high-powered professional or businessperson to take. I know because of my tendency to be a "control freak." But I've learned over the years that if I try to keep a finger in every pie, I quickly run out of fingers and have no time for a creative life of my own.

In the last analysis, every accomplished, successful person faces a paradox: Great individual success requires great trust in others. The farther we move up the ladder, the more we have to rely on the help and advice of others. In our increasingly specialized society, we must encourage others to fulfill responsibilities and perform tasks that we don't have the time, energy, or ability to do. Persons who fail to honor this basic work paradox are destined not only to be overwhelmed by bad stress, but also to be less productive, happy, and successful than if they just let go.

Travel

People who travel frequently, as I do, know that the time in transit always involves stress. But the bad stress can be transformed into a highly productive work time—and can even afford a welcome break from the trials and tribulations of daily work. The trick is to know how to minimize the stress and maximize the work efficiency and personal enjoyment.

Here are some tips I've picked up from the three to four months I spend traveling every year, as well as from other sources:

Tip #1: Always carry at least 50 percent more work than you feel you should reasonably be able to complete while traveling.

For a busy executive, few things are more frustrating than being thrust into a situation where you can't work when you know you need to work. The uncertainty of air travel can be a major threat to your peace of mind—unless you take steps to protect yourself from the potential stress of taking a trip.

For example, if I take the exact amount of work I think I can do, assuming my travel time and connections proceed perfectly, I may end up twiddling my thumbs whenever a flight is canceled or delayed. So I figure out how much I think I can do if there are no hitches, and then I add 50 percent.

Mutual fund guru John Templeton also believes in carrying around reports, articles, or other educational reading matter with him in the pocket of his suit jacket or in a light valise. If he gets stuck on a delayed flight, or if someone is late to an appointment, he is sure to have plenty to do until he can resume his planned schedule. As a result, he never gets annoyed or anxious when people are late or his travel plans are upset. (See William Proctor, *The Templeton Touch* [Doubleday, 1983], pp. 91–2.)

Tip #2: Always carry something relaxing and enjoyable to read.

On a long trip, you certainly won't be able to work every moment you are on your plane, ship, or train. In addition to your work material, take along a popular book, magazine, or other light reading material. If your carrier is delayed—and if you don't want to work—you will have something to divert your attention from the delay or uncertainty of your arrival.

Remember the cognitive-behavioral technique of substitution or distraction: If you can substitute a nonstressful activity that can hold your attention, you will be less likely to focus on the stressor and be overcome by high anxiety.

Tip #3: Allow plenty of time to catch your plane or other carrier.

People who habitually arrive at the ticket counter at the last minute are *asking* for a stressful experience. If you get there a half hour to an hour early, you can always work, read, make phone calls, or occupy yourself in other productive ways while you are waiting to board.

Tip #4: Exercise while traveling.

When I'm on a plane, I always stand up and walk the aisles several times. There are usually nooks and crannies at the back of every plane where you can do some stretching. The more you move about during a trip, the less likely you will be to become stiff and fatigued.

Tip #5: Drink plenty of clear, nonalcoholic, noncaffeinated fluids.

Airline and other travel experts warn that dehydration from dry cabin air can become a problem for many travelers. Your agitation and bad stress levels can increase if you fail to eat and drink properly during a trip. Fruit juices and water are essential dietary requirements for most travelers, especially those on a long trip.

Stay away from alcohol and beverages containing caffeine. They have a tendency to dehydrate or operate as diuretics (i.e., they cause fluids to leave the body). Also, drinks containing sodium, such as colas and sodas, may increase swelling (edema) in the ankles and elsewhere, which some people suffer during long flights. (See *Car & Travel,* November-December 1995, p. 9.)

A side note: Traveling on vacations can be even more stressful than traveling for business. Busy executives and professionals are increasingly finding that vacation traveling is becoming so stressful that they prefer to spend their vacations at home!

A survey by the Wirthlin Group, an opinion research firm, revealed that 40 percent of the one thousand adults surveyed said they were more likely to spend their vacations at home now than they were five years ago. Similarly, when representatives of Hilton Hotels Corporation questioned Americans about their travel habits, they learned that almost 30 percent of those who earned more than $100,000 a year *disagreed* with this statement: "For a vacation to be real, it must be away from home." (See *The Wall Street Journal Report,* October 20, 1995, p. B1.)

Multitasking

Predictably, *multitasking* is a term introduced into the vocabulary of the business world by the computer and electronics industry. The word refers to the attempt to do several jobs or tasks at once—and often electronic gadgets are the means to that end.

A multitasking person might try to work simultaneously with a couple of phone conversations on different lines, a computer keyboard, a fax machine, and maybe even a beeper. The worst offenders probably also have a couple of clients waiting in the reception area while the electronic juggling is going on.

Psychologists are finding more and more often that they have to treat workers with this multitasking problem because the electronic tools that are supposed to make life easier are actually compounding the stress. Psychiatrists at the Harvard

Medical School who run executive seminars have reported that a session on technology-induced exhaustion is the most popular selection. (See *The Wall Street Journal,* April 19, 1995, p. B1.)

Those treating multitaskers find that not only does their stress increase, but so do the mistakes. The human brain has an immense capacity to do work, but paying only partial attention to a job can cause a worker to become distracted and perhaps put a crucial number in the wrong column.

A more insidious threat is "creep" in your work hours. If you are always accessible by cellular phone, beeper, fax, or other devices, you are in effect always at work. Your leisure time, including time with your family, will never be true quality time. All this leads to overwork—and in our discussion of workload, we've seen the health threat that can pose.

Besides exacerbating general stress and interfering with relationships, multitasking can be dangerous to your health in other ways. The National Highway Traffic Safety Administration has announced that it has begun tracking data on accidents related to cellular phone use on the roads.

What's the antidote to multitasking? The only answer is to cut back on multitasking. Don't try to handle several electronic devices at once. Don't talk on the phone while you drive. Delegate some of your tasks to others. The sense of power, control, and increased efficiency you think you are getting from multitasking is really an illusion. The human brain just isn't designed to operate this way!

There are plenty of other possible sources for burnout on the job, including office politics and impossible bosses. You can undoubtedly add your own special stressors to this list. But whatever the reason for your job stress, several responses have been applied successfully to almost every conceivable situation. These constitute the Paradox Prescription for burnout.

The Paradox Prescription for Burnout

Your response to burnout, and job stress in general, begins with the two basic paradoxes we explored at the beginning of this chapter: release and retreat. But beyond these fundamental principles, specific techniques have been established through research or clinical experience as quite useful in dealing with on-the-job pressure. Let's consider some of the most potent "prescriptions."

Assertiveness

As a general rule, remaining passive in a stressful situation tends to *raise* levels of bad stress. In contrast, taking steps to be more assertive and active in dealing with stressors can reduce stress levels.

For example, executives I treat who are displaying serious signs of stress often tend to be characterized by an unwillingness to talk to the oppressive boss or confront the obnoxious coworker who may be responsible for the stressful reaction.

On the other hand, those who are willing to assert themselves in a rational, low-key fashion—without allowing themselves to become angry or overly aggressive—tend to handle stress on the job much better.

You'll recall my experience on board the ship during Typhoon Zane, which I described in the very first chapter of this book. In part, I succeeded in keeping my stress levels low during that crisis by asserting myself with the ship's staff, but without letting my emotions get the best of me.

Similarly, in a 1994 study of the effectiveness of assertiveness training among sixty nurses in Taiwan, Republic of China, researchers divided the subjects into two groups. One was assigned to assertiveness training, and a control group was given unrelated instruction in computers. Both groups participated in six two-hour workshops during the same two-week period. Also, both turned in low scores on an assertiveness pretest, and both were evaluated as being under considerable stress at work.

At the end of the study, the assertiveness training group scored significantly higher on a psychological test for assertiveness than did those in the control group. Also, the assertiveness group reported significantly lower levels of stress than the controls. The investigators concluded that the results clearly support the effectiveness of assertiveness training for treating nonassertive behavior and high stress among the nurses. (See *Issues of Mental Health in Nursing,* July-August 1994, pp. 419–32.)

Control

An issue that is closely related to healthy assertiveness is the exercise of personal control over a stressful situation. In other words, if you can maintain a certain degree of control over your work life—either through assertiveness or some other means—you are much less likely to become stressed out.

Greek scientists at the Nursing Department, University of Athens, explored whether nurses specializing in cancer patients (oncology nurses) experience higher levels of burnout than nurses working in general hospitals. In particular, the researchers looked into the effect of personal and environmental factors on emotional exhaustion, a sense of depersonalization, and a lack of personal accomplishment.

After comparing 217 nurses in oncological hospitals with 226 nurses in general hospitals, the investigators found no statistical difference in burnout in the two groups. But they did find that a sense of personal control in individual nurses was the major factor that protected them from emotional exhaustion, depersonalization, and a lack of personal accomplishment. (See *British Journal of Medical Psychology,* June 1994, pp. 187–99.)

A lack of personal control can have various serious health effects, including an impact on the health of unborn children. Scientists at the Department of Gynecology and Obstetrics, Aarhus University Hospital, Denmark, evaluated 8,711 pregnant Danish women between 1989 and 1991. The purpose was to check the impact of job demands and control on pregnancy risk and size of newborns.

First, they divided the women into four "exposure categories": (1) relaxed jobs (low demands, high control); (2) active jobs (high demands, high control); (3) passive jobs (low demands, low control); and (4) high-strain jobs (high demands, low control). Then, they evaluated the outcome of their pregnancies.

The results? Those with relaxed jobs (low demands, high control) had the lowest risk of abnormally small babies and of premature delivery. Also, though the numbers were too small to be "statistically significant," they found that all risks increased consistently with low job control. (See *International Journal of Epidemiology,* August 1994, pp. 764–74.)

Planning

A carefully planned schedule or work plan may cut two ways: If you try to adhere to it too rigidly, you may increase your bad stress levels as inevitable glitches and changes occur in your plan. On the other hand, if you use your plan more as a guide, with the understanding that the uncertainties of life will make adjustments inevitable, a plan can be a useful tool in minimizing stress.

One practical example I recommend is making to-do lists. Busy people who get into the habit of using such lists almost always find that they are less likely to have a sense of confusion or "loose ends" in their daily schedules.

The reason is that if you have eight or ten things to do and you put them down on paper, you find immediate relief because you don't have to hold them in your mind. You can, in effect, forget the whole list as you tend to a particular item because you know that when you finish that item, you can return to the list to see what comes up next. Also, the list provides a sense of control: You have a plan, represented by the list, and you can exercise control by checking off each item after you finish it.

A related technique worked with hospital workers studied by the Care Research and Development Unit, University of Lund, Sweden. These people, who worked with severely demented patients, were divided into two groups. One was given a carefully designed patient plan and systematic supervision. The other control group received no special help in their work.

At the end of the study, the group with the plan and supervision experienced considerably lower stress levels. Also, their creativity on the job increased. (See *Journal of Advanced Nursing*, October 1994, pp. 742–9.)

Relaxation Techniques

We've already seen in some detail in Chapter 6 how relaxation training can lower stress levels. Everything that was said in that context also applies to lowering the levels of job stress and the risk of burnout. But I want to make an additional point about relaxation training that may be of some interest to the athletically minded.

A study was done at John Carroll University in Cleveland, Ohio, to compare the effectiveness of relaxation training versus the use of mental imagery techniques on the accuracy of basketball foul shooting. The investigators pretested eighteen female college basketball players, who were then assigned alternately to relaxation or mental imagery training. They were tested again after four training sessions per week for three weeks.

Contrary to expectations, the imagery group did not improve. But the group using relaxation techniques turned in a marginally superior performance in foul shooting. (See *Perception and Motor Skills*, June 1994, pp. 1229–30.)

Special "Retreat" Responses

Sometimes, the only effective way to deal with job stress and impending burnout is to get away from the job. Unless I take off one day a week—and plan several short holidays or vacations during the year—my bad stress levels become unbearable.

In a study of Canadian emergency room physicians, researchers measured their stress levels through several established psychological scales. They found that 46 percent fell within the medium to high levels of emotional exhaustion; 93 percent were within the medium to high range for depersonalization; and 79 percent were in the medium to low range for personal accomplishment.

Those who were most satisfied with their work were older and were heads of departments, and they were in the habit of taking long holidays each year. On the other hand, factors associated with *lower* job satisfaction were involvement in medical education and increased clinical hours worked. The researchers concluded that time away from clinical practice is important to job satisfaction and emotional well-being. (See *Journal of Emergency Medicine,* July-August 1994, pp. 559–65.)

Some other ways of retreating from work are more radical—though worth consideration. For one thing, observers of the work scene have noted that increasing numbers of people seem to be *downshifting.* This may include switching to a less stressful job, cutting back drastically on workload, or picking up new, creative interests (such as taking adult education courses or getting more involved in volunteer or church activities).

Usually, as work researcher and economist Juliet Schor has pointed out, the *down* in this term means down in income and also down in the stress and pace of life. In her research for her 1993 book *The Overworked American* (Basic Books), Schor found that 28 percent of eight hundred American adults whom she and the Merck Family Fund surveyed acknowledged downshifting in some way. (See *Harvard Magazine,* September-October 1995, pp. 12–3.)

In the same vein, the Trends Research Institute of Rhinebeck, New York, has pinpointed "voluntary simplicity" as one of its top ten trends of the 1990s. This group predicts that by the end of the decade, 15 percent of America's 77 million baby boomers will be part of a "simplicity" market for various home gardening and other consumer products related to the simpler life.

Support of these predictions can be found in other research. The Harwood Group of Bethesda, Maryland, released a study in 1995 that showed 82 percent of Americans believe we buy and consume far more than we need. Also, 28 percent had voluntarily taken a pay cut in the last five years, and 86 percent of all downshifters reported feeling "happy" about their changes in jobs and circumstances. (See *The New York Times,* September 21, 1995, p. B1.)

These and other findings by various scientists and other researchers have established beyond any doubt that job stress has become an epidemic in our society. Yet many effective responses are available. Your challenge is to consider the possibilities that have been listed in this chapter and see which ones may reduce stress levels and risk of burnout in your life. Use what you have read as a kind of checklist, and feel free to add other stress antidotes that may come to mind.

Then, act! Don't let another day go by without drafting your own Paradox Prescription to relieve stress—as well as unhappiness and low productivity—in your work environment.

CHAPTER 8

WHY YOU SHOULD RELAX
IN YOUR RELATIONSHIPS

Good relationships are rooted in conflict. In fact, it's impossible to achieve harmony in any relationship without the presence of conflict.

This paradox underlies many of the principles and recommendations in this chapter, but how can it be true? Isn't the main feature of a good relationship the *absence* of conflict? And won't interpersonal conflict of any kind increase your levels of negative stress?

The solution to this paradox involves understanding the real nature of the conflict that goes into a good relationship. You should shoot for *controlled* conflict—and especially, a successful resolution of that conflict. This means achieving the freedom to disagree, argue, and confront, yet to do so in such a way that words and actions don't turn into weapons of destruction.

As low-grade conflict follows its course, the people involved must assume—must *know*—that the relationship itself never depends on the outcome of any particular confrontation or argument. Rather, the ultimate objective of controlled conflict is to test weak points in a relationship so that they become stronger and stronger, much as steel becomes stronger in the refining fires of a furnace.

Let me give you a personal example. My wife, Millie, and I frequently disagree on practically any topic you can imagine. An outsider overhearing one of our conversations might wonder, *How on earth did those two ever get together—and how do they stay together?*

The answer is easy: We got together because from the beginning, we found each other's company challenging and stimulating. When I take a new intellectual, political, or theological position with Millie, I know I have to be ready to defend it or go down in flames if I don't have good arguments to back up my opinion.

At the same time, we are completely confident that our marriage doesn't depend on the outcome of any particular discussion. Rather, we have learned over many years that controlled conflict is the spice of life—an enjoyable kind of positive stress that binds us closer as husband and wife.

I believe this same principle applies to all relationships. Whether you are dealing with children, parents, siblings, or friends, conflict cannot and should not be avoided. But it can and must be controlled—as scientific studies are now beginning to demonstrate.

In a 1992 study of married couples by University of Utah psychologists, published in *Health Psychology,* husbands were asked to persuade their wives to change their minds on a particular topic. The husbands, who got angry, displayed a marked rise in blood pressure as they tried to make their point. But wives who took on the persuader role didn't become as angry, and their blood pressure measurements were unaffected. On the other hand, in a related study at Johns Hopkins University, couples who learned and abided by some rules of fair fighting found that blood pressure actually declined in hypertensive husbands. (See *The New York Times,* December 15, 1992, pp. C1, C12.)

In effect, a relationship that is based on constructive, controlled conflict is a relationship that is "relaxed." By this, I mean that the relationship is filled with good, rather than bad, stress. Confrontations, arguments, and clashes become enjoyable and diverting as they build, rather than tear down, personal connections, both in the present and in the future.

To understand how this works, we'll first consider what may happen when conflict and bad stress in a relationship get out of control. Then, we'll explore ways to eliminate the bad stress.

The Medical Rationale for Relaxed Relationships

If conflict gets out of control in a close relationship, especially a family relationship, the typical medical symptoms of bad stress may not be far behind.

I recall observing some classic symptoms in a forty-year-old man whose marriage was falling apart. I had last seen him when he and his wife were still together. On that occasion, he was athletic looking, walked with an easy swagger, and seemed closer to thirty than forty.

When I saw him again after he had been separated from his wife for a couple of months, I almost didn't recognize him. He had lost at least fifteen pounds—undoubtedly due to the loss of appetite that often accompanies emotional depression. His face appeared haunted and his eyes watery, a signal that he wasn't sleeping well. He carried himself stiffly, almost like an old man. As it turned out, he had "thrown his back out" soon after his wife departed. He had just come down with the flu—a sign that his immune system was not working properly. Beyond these common signs and symptoms of heavy stress, a difficult relationship may trigger much more serious problems.

The Cardiovascular Connection

For example, a 1995 presentation on stress for the American Heart Association by Lisa Berkman, an epidemiologist at Yale University School of Medicine, showed that people who are isolated from family or friends following a heart attack are three times more likely to die than other heart attack sufferers.

Other studies have established that married men have a lower risk of dying young than single men. Also, according to a 1988 review in *Science,* people with few friends or family relations have a death rate from two to four times as great as those with many personal connections.

Reporting on research she has done at the molecular level, Dr. Berkman noted that emotional support from others can alter an individual's levels of norepinephrine and cortisol, the adrenal hormones that may circulate in the brain. These chemicals are believed to affect blood pressure and the general responses of the heart to stress.

Dr. Berkman concluded that if you are convinced that you have emotional support from others, your body may be less vulnerable to bad stress. Specifically, your blood pressure and heart rate will stay lower. She defined emotional support as being with a loved one or friend, talking with the other person, and helping that person make decisions. (See Associated Press release, January 19, 1995.)

Asthma—Again

As we saw in Chapter 2, asthma may be another end result of serious family stress and conflict, especially in crowded urban settings. In fact, asthma, with irritation of the bronchial passages that impedes breathing, increased by 34 percent from 1983 to 1993, according to the National Institutes of Health. (See *The New York Times,* September 1995, pp. A1, A14.)

The Bowel Response

Still another possible result of family or other relational conflict is irritable bowel disease. (This syndrome, which may

---

afflict as many as one-fifth of the adult American population, involves an ongoing series of gastrointestinal symptoms, including regular stomach pains and recurrent alterations in the frequency of bowel movements.)

According to the Department of Medicine, University of Sydney, Nepean Hospital, Australia, there may be a link between functional bowel disease and sexual, physical, emotional, or verbal abuse. The researchers evaluated 997 patients and found that those who have been abused are significantly more likely to report irritable bowel symptoms than those who do not report being abused. (See *American Journal of Gastroenterology,* March 1995, pp. 366–71.)

Obviously, the source of heart disease, asthma, and irritable bowel syndrome may be traced to influences other than stress. But in many cases, bad stress—including relational stress—seems to play a major role.

This observation, in turn, brings us to a fundamental question: What factors may cause conflicts to get out of control and trigger serious health symptoms? In many cases, the problems begin and end with uncontrolled anger.

A Prescription That Begins and Ends with Anger

In 1992, when he was fifty-three years old, Lance Morrow, a senior writer at *Time,* was hit with his second heart attack. His search for the reasons for his health problems led him to conclude in his book, *Heart: A Memoir* (Warner Books, 1995), that the cause of his health problems was the rage he had inherited from his mother, including periodic bursts of anger that would flare up "like a bucket of gasoline thrown on a campfire." (See *The New York Times,* September 15, 1995, p. B8.)

After studying the records of thousands of patients at the Cooper Clinic, I have come to a similar conclusion: More often than not, simmering anger lies behind much of today's negative stress. The feelings typically begin with frustration or irritation at someone or some situation. Then, the hostility intensifies until it turns into full-blown, chronic anger.

The public perception is that our society is growing angrier by the minute. According to a survey conducted by the *Dallas Morning News* (August 20, 1995, p. 1), 69 percent of the adults who responded felt that people are angrier than they were a few years ago. About 50 percent of those polled said they got angry at least once a week while driving or while watching or reading the news. More than 33 percent got angry at least once a week at work or at home.

The impact of such ongoing anger on health can be devastating. A 1996 study published in *Circulation* by Dr. Ichiro Kawachi and others at the Harvard School of Public Health found that men who scored highest on a standard anger scale were three times as likely to suffer heart disease during a seven-year period as those who scored lowest in anger. (See *The New York Times,* November 20, 1996, p. B9.)

Such observations have convinced me that any effort to develop more productive relationships with others must often begin and end with anger. In other words, we must find the source of the angry "fires" inside us, as Lance Morrow would say, and then put them out.

But when you finally identify the source of your anger, what can you do to overcome it?

In the *Dallas Morning News* survey just mentioned, the respondents gave interesting practical responses they have found helpful in dealing with their anger. Here are some of the more promising ideas:

- 84 percent said they "talk to someone."
- 76 percent "pray."
- 67 percent "take a deep breath or count to 10."
- 58 percent "take a walk."
- 52 percent "exercise or participate in a sport."

How well do these responses work?

Scientific studies seem to back up some of these survey findings. For example, as a result of research with more than four hundred men and women, aged sixteen to seventy-five, Dr. Diane Tice, a psychologist at Case Western University, in Cleveland, Ohio, reports that going for long walks is often a good antidote for anger. Also, it helps to step back or detach yourself from your hostile feelings and try to see the situation from the other person's viewpoint. In addition, taking some time to cool off before you try to talk to an offensive person can be an effective strategy. On the other hand, reacting immediately, such as by launching a personal angry attack on the other person, doesn't help your inner tranquillity or the relationship. (See *The New York Times,* December 30, 1992, p. C6.)

It has even been suggested that dietary measures may lessen anger and hostility in some people. In one 1992 study conducted at the State University of New York at Stony Brook, families that switched to a diet low in fat and high in complex carbohydrates (such as fruits and vegetables) began to display lower levels of hostility in their relationships. They also experienced reduced levels of depression and blood cholesterol. (See *The New York Times,* November 20, 1996, p. B9.)

Although one or more of these coping mechanisms may help you counter the anger that leads to excessive stress, some other responses are almost certain to *increase* the stress that comes from anger. Other groups of respondents in the newspaper survey just cited, for instance, reported these responses to their feelings of anger:

- 57 percent "swear or curse."
- 46 percent "scream or yell."
- 33 percent "eat."
- 16 percent "drink alcohol."
- 6 percent "throw or break something."
- 3 percent "hit someone."

Such reactions are certainly natural and common. But avoid them at all costs! They will either add fuel to your emotional fires and make your anger worse than ever, or cause serious harm to your mind and body.

A Stanford University study (published in August 1992 in the *American Journal of Cardiology*) reported that the pumping efficiency of the heart is reduced when a person becomes angry. Just venting anger or blowing up can make the emotion grow stronger, according to Dr. Gail Ironson, a psychiatrist who headed the research.

On the other hand, she doesn't think you should try to suppress your anger or hold it in. Rather, it's best to express it with controlled assertiveness—such as by calmly discussing your feelings and concerns with the person who is the target of your anger. (See *The New York Times*, September 2, 1992, p. C12.)

To sum up, then, I suggest that first, you do some soul-searching to determine whether or not you really are angry about something. Then, the next step is to find out what is causing the hostility and begin to deal with it aggressively.

Let's suppose the source of your anger and conflict can be traced to your marriage and family life. What might be the specific nature of the problem, and what should you do about it?

The Special Stress of Marriage

A considerable body of research establishes the fact that a strong marriage—with controlled conflict—can benefit both spouses.

According to demographic findings presented at the conference of the Population Association of America in San Francisco on April 8, 1995, marriage offers significant emotional, financial, and health benefits. Divorced men, for instance, were reported to have twice the rate of alcohol abuse of married men. Also, married people have more and better sex than single people, according to a 1992 National Health and Social Life survey cited at the conference.

Overall, men seem to benefit more from marriage than women—though married couples were found to be generally better off financially than couples who merely lived together.

In general, the demographers at the conference argued against cohabitation on several grounds. They said that those who live together before marriage have higher divorce rates and are more likely to be sexually unfaithful and self-centered than those who start out their relationship in marriage. (See *The New York Times*, April 10, 1995, p. A8.)

As all married people know, getting along with a spouse isn't always easy. Because you tend to spend more time with your spouse than with anyone else, the opportunities for stress are magnified in marriage.

In studies conducted by immunologists at the Ohio State University Medical School, ninety couples were placed in a laboratory where they were directed to resolve a disagreement in their marriage. Steady blood monitoring for a twenty-four-hour period revealed that the couples with the most hostility and negativity during the interactions experienced a broad drop in their immune responses. The researchers concluded that the more hostile you are during a marital argument, the harder it is on your immune system. (See *The New York Times*, December 15, 1992, pp. C1, C12.)

In a related Ohio State University study of older couples, presented in 1996 at the International Congress of Behavioral Medicine, the researchers found that marital fights can weaken the immune systems of couples who have been happily married for many years.

The study, which involved thirty-one older couples, aged fifty-five to seventy-five, revealed that stress hormones rose with the arguments. Specifically, three of these hormones—ACTH, norepinephrine, and cortisol—increased as the conflict increased. The stress hormones stayed higher than normal for at least fifteen minutes after the arguments ended. The most significant rises in hormones occurred among the female participants. (See report from *The Washington Post,* published in *The Palm Beach Post,* May 14, 1996, p. 3D.)

What About the Children?

In general, stress in the family arises from excessive conflict, not the configuration of the family or the ages of the spouses.

In a 1995 review article produced at the Department of Psychiatry, Stanford University, scientists noted that the shift from traditional family forms (i.e., the nuclear family) has been dramatic. Only an estimated 50 percent of children will live with their biologic parents until their eighteenth birthday.

The research also indicated that it is not the form of the family, but conflict that produces lasting emotional difficulties in the children. (See *Pediatric Clinics of North America,* February 1995, pp. 31–43.)

In a study at the Department of Pediatrics, Vanderbilt University School of Medicine, Nashville, Tennessee, researchers examined the impact of "negative life events" on 197 children with chronic abdominal pain. The negative life events included school and social problems and sexual abuse.

The researchers found that boys who came from families with many negative life events—and whose mothers had physical complaints—had more physical problems. (See *Journal of Consulting Clinical Psychology,* December 1994, vol. 62, pp. 1213–21.)

The ultimate result from family conflict ending in divorce may even be an early death for the children. The seventy-seven-year-old Terman study has tracked those who achieved very high scores (135 and above) on the Stanford-Binet IQ test. The investigators reported in 1995 that those children whose parents were divorced have faced a 33 percent greater risk of an earlier death than those whose parents remained married until the children reached age twenty-one. (See *The New York Times,* March 7, 1995, p. B5.)

So what can we conclude about family stress from these findings? Here are a few suggestions:

- Spouses should feel free to engage in arguments and conflict, but only when clear ground rules have been established to control and resolve the disagreements.
- To maximize health and happiness, choose marriage over cohabitation.

- Children may be the main health casualties of uncontrolled marital conflict and divorce—so parents should do all they can to shield their offspring from exposure to excessive conflict. On the other hand, teaching a child by example how to resolve family conflicts successfully may not only enhance the child's current well-being, but may also provide a valuable model for the child's future marriage.

An Epilogue on Elder Care

As the demographics of our society shift and the older population becomes proportionally larger, the focus has been moving more toward the needs of elderly people—and especially ways families can care for their older members.

The stress in these changes may cut two ways: against both the younger caregiver and the aging family member, who must confront shrinking resources, deteriorating health, and emotional problems, especially depression.

Stress Among the Caregivers

If a younger family member decides to take responsibility for the care of a parent or other elderly relative, the administrative and logistical challenges can be overwhelming. Many adult children have found themselves embarking on a full-time job as they attempt to become instant experts on Medicare and Medicaid requirements, investments and other financial matters, health concerns, nursing homes, and the like.

The most stressful kind of elder care is long-distance caregiving, or being one who cares for an elderly relative who lives miles away. Estimates published in *The Wall Street Journal* (October 18, 1995, p. B1) indicated that 12 to 15 percent of workers currently provide elder care, and 2 to 6 percent of workers care for elders who live more than an hour away.

How can you reduce your stress levels if you are caring for an aging and infirm relative?

There are no easy answers, but many of the techniques already discussed for reducing stress are applicable. To begin with, you can increase your sense of control by formulating an overall strategy or plan to help your relative. Also, commit your plan to paper because there are likely to be too many details and possibilities to try to carry everything around in your head.

Obviously, since you are moving into uncharted waters with the prospect of constantly changing health, living arrangements, and financial needs, you can't expect to write your plan in concrete. You are bound to encounter changes as you move along. But just having an overall strategy on paper at the outset will do wonders to reduce your stress levels.

Then, with your plan in hand, you should take the initiative and become assertive in following the strategy you have selected. Be disciplined! Under no circumstances should you try to "shoot from the hip" by responding to crises as they appear. If you take this chaotic approach, you will almost certainly be totally confused, out of control, and in the grips of unbearable stress.

After you have drawn up your plan, gather as many written sources as you can from agencies and other organizations. For example, if you are concerned about home nursing care, check your local library and bookstore for sources, and above all, call the local hospital. If your problems are primarily legal, you may want to find an attorney who specializes in the new field of "elderlaw"—and gather booklets and brochures to bring you up to speed on the subject.

Once you have read through the relevant sources, you will undoubtedly want to make adjustments in your written plan. Then, proceed to make the personal contacts you will need to move toward a solution for your elderly relative.

Admittedly, these suggestions are rather sketchy because this book's focus is not on the care of elderly relatives. But the principles of stress management should be familiar: Make a plan. Write it down. Be systematic and assertive in following the plan. Don't be surprised when the plan has to be altered because of changing circumstances and information.

All these points may seem self-evident, but I'm amazed at how many people plunge into a complex issue like elder care without formulating an overall strategy and following it. As you know, there is ample scientific support for these "self-evident" steps to get the job done at a manageable level of stress. Too often, we forget to follow the obvious path, and high levels of bad stress result.

Stress Among Elderly People

Even as you pursue an intelligent and reasonable strategy to care for your older relative, you may fail unless you understand what that older man or woman is going through.

First of all, don't assume you are dealing with the same mother, father, aunt, or uncle you knew twenty or thirty years ago. Time and bad health may have caused changes in the ability to think clearly and react well to difficult circumstances. Older people typically become fearful about their condition and the future. Also, chemical changes in the brain that often occur with aging may cause many older people to become depressed.

The National Institute on Aging has compiled a list of common signs of depression in elderly people, including the following:

- Fatigue and lack of energy
- An "empty" feeling
- Ongoing sadness and anxiety
- Loss of interest in ordinary activities, including sex
- Sleep problems
- Eating problems—either loss of appetite or increase in appetite
- Constant crying
- Irritability
- Thoughts that drift to suicide or death
- Chronic aches and pains
- Problems with memory or concentration

• Pessimism about the future

If you see any of these signs in the elderly person you are caring for, you should seek medical help. Among other things, depression among men and women sixty-five and older has been found to nearly triple the risk of a stroke. (See *The New York Times*, September 6, 1995, p. B6.)

As we have moved through this book, the medical implications of bad stress have become more and more apparent. With stress, we are not just talking about an emotional or psychological phenomenon, but a force that can severely damage the body and even cut short the life span. Yet to find out where you stand physically in the face of your stressful life, you need something more than what we have discussed so far. Read on to learn about practical guidelines that can turn your regular medical exam into a "stress checkup."

CHAPTER 9

DECIPHERING YOUR BODY'S STRESS STATUS

If you listen to your body when you are under stress, it will speak to you in a still, small voice or in loud, clear tones. It's up to you to listen and respond, either by taking preventive measures on your own—such as altering your diet or exercise regimen—or by consulting your physician.

This brings us to the seventh and final step in the Paradox Prescription: seeing your doctor for regular "stress checkups." Here is how this extremely important process works:

When you begin to feel the weight of bad stress, you can be sure that your body will start sending you messages. You must be alert to pick up the first signals about your physical and emotional health, including your stress status. Then, be prepared to act appropriately.

You make the doctor's job easier when you provide details about what your body has been saying. The stressed-out patients who come through my offices say,

- "I'm always tired."
- "I have frequent backaches."
- "I have trouble sleeping."
- "I'm having trouble concentrating, and my memory seems off the mark."
- "I seem to be losing my sex drive."
- "I often get headaches, apparently for no reason."
- "My stomach is frequently upset."
- "My bowels are unpredictable; sometimes I'm constipated, and other times my stool is loose."

Receiving this input from my patients is extremely helpful. Among other things, their observations about themselves give me special guidance about where to focus my attention—whether on a stress-related matter or in another direction.

Of course, regardless of the information the patient conveys, I conduct a complete medical exam, and sometimes, this general checkup will reveal a problem that the patient wasn't aware of. But often, the alert patient will pick up signals that make it possible to identify and treat medical problems at a very early stage.

Early diagnosis and speedy treatment of disease are two essential components of a long and vigorous life. It doesn't help to be aerobically fit, strong, and flexible—and at the same time to be suffering from a disease that threatens health or life. The medical exam and an ability to listen to your particular body's language and respond when warning bells begin to ring are the cornerstones for any successful stress-management program.

Some basic "rules of wellness" will help you make the best use of your physician. The first rule is to be faithful in having a regular checkup. The second rule is to be firm in demanding from your doctor the seven essential exams that every adult should have at the scheduled checkup. The third rule says that you should have near at hand a list of the proven treatments available for the most common stress-related complaints.

Wellness Rule #1: Be Religious About Your Medical Exam

Probably the most important mistake made by the running guru Jim Fixx, author of the best-seller *The Complete Book of Running*, is that he neglected to have regular medical exams, including stress tests with exercise electrocardiograms. His failure to go in for a regular checkup was a key ingredient in his early death at age fifty-two. A stress test would almost certainly have picked up the blocked coronary arteries that led to his fatal heart attack. With that information, Fixx and his physicians could most likely have saved his life.

To avoid the Fixx fallacy, you should undergo a complete medical-wellness exam with your physician. (A detailed description of such an exam can be found in my book *The Aerobics Program for Total Well-Being* [Bantam, 1983], pp. 219ff.) Here are some guidelines for timing the exam:

- Everyone under age forty should have at least one complete physical, which will serve as a baseline or standard for later exams.
- People aged forty to fifty should have a thorough physical, including a stress test, *every year to eighteen months.* Women should undergo a mammography during these exams. Every two years during this period, both men and women should have a colon exam using a proctosigmoidoscope (a long, rigid or flexible device, which is inserted 25 to 60 centimeters into the large intestine through the rectum so that the doctor can view the walls of the colon).
- People aged fifty and older should have an *annual* physical with stress electrocardiogram and mammography, and every two years, they should also have a proctosigmoidoscope exam, and every five years a barium enema or colonoscopy.

These are just basic ground rules about medical exams, but what about specific conditions that may be directly related to stress? Let's consider some that your doctor may identify.

Common Stress-Related Physical Problems

The following serious conditions, which stress may trigger or aggravate, can pose a major threat to your health or life. A complete physical exam is designed to pick these up early if you make regular appointments with your doctor:

- Heart disease
- Cancer
- Hypertension
- Osteoporosis and other bone diseases
- Diabetes

Anytime you miss one of your regular exams, you increase your health risks. If one of these conditions is present, it will most likely worsen with additional time and inattention. Pursuing a good diet, engaging in regular exercise, and taking other preventive measures just aren't enough to afford complete protection from serious disease. Remember, absolutely essential components for good health are early diagnosis and speedy treatment of disease. The annual medical exam facilitates your achievement of these objectives.

Wellness Rule #2: Request the Seven Essential "Stress Checkup" Exams

This section emphasizes seven exams that I regard as essential during your regular physical. Each will not only enable your doctor to check the impact of excessive stress, but will also help him or her monitor your general health more effectively.

Of course, I'm *not* saying that these are the only tests you need during your annual checkup. I just want to alert you first of all to the fact that they are among the most important. Also, you should be aggressive in requesting them because not all physicians will provide all of the tests and procedures—at least not unless you ask for them.

For example, only a few doctors have treadmills or other stress test equipment available in their examining rooms. If you request this test, they will have to send you to another clinic. Many will not even suggest the test unless you ask for it.

Similarly, some doctors do not like to do the proctosigmoidoscope exam. Instead, they may refer you to a specialist, even though this particular procedure is well within the capability of a qualified internist.

As for blood tests, many doctors provide you only with a total cholesterol measurement—not the all-important subcomponents, including the "good" (HDL) cholesterol and the "bad" (LDL) cholesterol. Nor will they automatically test your triglyceride levels or give the homocysteine test, both of which have recently gained significance as ways of evaluating the risk of heart disease.

For ease of memory, you can divide the seven essential tests into two main stress checkup categories: the Cardiovascular Check and the Cancer Check. Again, keep in mind that the following is intended only as an overview, not a complete treatment of the details and measurement categories of each test. That information is available in my other books.

The Cardiovascular Check

This first category involves evaluations for heart disease, stroke risk, and other cardiovascular problems.

1. The stress test. A treadmill test is best, but a stationary bicycle may be used if the patient cannot perform on the treadmill. The test involves first taking a resting electrocardiogram (EKG), with at least ten electrodes (rubber patches attached to EKG wires) on the chest. Fewer electrodes or leads will greatly increase the tendency toward errors.

Then, using the treadmill, you are given an exercise electrocardiogram. The objective is to exercise to exhaustion, or until you reach your predicted maximal heart rate. Stopping before exhaustion will limit the value of the test and may allow hidden heart disease to escape notice.

2. A complete blood and urine workup, including measurement of total cholesterol, cholesterol subcomponents (HDL and LDL), and other blood lipids. Remember that excessive stress can affect the balance of various components in your blood. For example, heavy bad stress can cause your cholesterol count to rise. Also, your white blood cell count may be affected as your immune function comes under attack.

A common blood test used by many good clinics is known as the SMAC-20 because twenty different blood studies are involved. In addition, you should ask for the homocysteine test, which is now given only rarely as a standard part of an annual physical, but which is effective in evaluating the risk of heart disease and other health problems.

3. Blood pressure monitoring. Every doctor should perform a blood pressure exam as a matter of routine. This test—along with treatments to control high blood pressure—is especially important to reduce the risk for stroke.

The Cancer Check

The second main category for your annual stress checkup provides you with several essential cancer tests.

4. Bowel tests. The basic procedure to check for possible cancer in the intestines is the fecal occult blood test. This self-administered exam requires collecting three samples of stool over a three-day period. Traces of blood in the samples can help your physician detect possible cancers or other types of bleeding somewhere in the gastrointestinal tract.

The second important intestinal exam is the proctosigmoidoscopy, involving the insertion into the colon of a rigid (or flexible) snakelike tube, which may measure 25 or 60 centimeters. The 60-centimeter scope will detect almost two-thirds of lesions or cancers in the colon, while the 25-centimeter device will detect somewhat fewer.

Note: Another test, called a "colonoscopy," involves the use of a long colonoscope, which can cover the entire length of the colon. Although this exam requires more time, it is sometimes referred to as the "gold standard" for screening cancer of the large intestine.

Some physicians who don't want to bother with one of these extensive colon exams may check your rectum and lower colon with a gloved finger. But this technique enables them to detect only 10 to 13 percent of cancers of the colon or rectum. Because of these limitations, this method should not be regarded as adequate by itself.

5. The prostate exam for men. Prostate cancer is the second greatest cause of cancer mortality in American men, with lung cancer being first. Cancer of the prostate has increased from 17,772 deaths in 1971 to 41,400 deaths in 1996, and it seems to be occurring at younger ages.

These symptoms may signal a prostate problem:

- Weak or interrupted flow of urine
- Inability to urinate or difficulty in starting urination
- A need to urinate frequently, especially at night
- Blood in the urine
- Urine flow that cannot be stopped easily
- Painful or burning sensation during urination
- Continuing pain in the lower back, pelvis, or upper thighs

If you have any of these symptoms, see your physician right away. But even if you don't have symptoms, you should still have a prostate check as part of your annual exam. That's the best way to head off any problem.

Be sure to ask for the blood test for prostate cancer, the Prostate Specific Antigen (PSA). The normal range for men

40 to 49 years old is 0 to 2.5; for men 50 to 59, 0 to 3.5; for men 60 to 69, 0 to 4.5; and for men 70 and older, 0 to 6.5. Values above 8.0 strongly suggest a problem.

6. Mammography for women. To check for cancer of the breast, the mammography exam should be given at least every two years to women fourty to fifty years of age. Women over fifty should take the exam annually.

7. The Pap test and a complete pelvic exam. These must be part of a woman's annual visit to the gynecologist because they are musts to detect early cancer in women.

As I've said, these seven tests aren't the only ones that should be part of a complete physical for adults, but they tend to be key tests for evaluating the impact of stress. Furthermore, one or more of these tests are likely to be omitted by many physicians during an annual physical.

I recommend that you jot them down on a slip of paper and take the list with you to your doctor's office just so you can be sure no important test is left out.

Wellness Rule #3: Don't Overlook the "Little" Stress Complaints

When you go in to see your doctor for your annual physical, you will probably be most concerned about "big" items, such as heart disease and cancer. If you receive a clean bill of health, your tendency may be to give a sigh of relief and get out of the doctor's office as fast as you can.

But don't be too hasty. It will be wonderful news to hear you are not suffering from a serious disease. However, a number of "little" complaints, all related to excessive stress, can make life miserable if you don't learn to care for them. Your physician is the expert to turn to for advice about the small problems that can loom large in daily life.

Three "little" complaints that I have found to be among the most common for those suffering from excessive stress are chronic fatigue, back pain, and insomnia. These concerns may make it unpleasant or even impossible to pursue an active life. Yet it's essential to not become discouraged when one of these minor conditions strikes. Rather, you should have a plan in mind to deal with the problem swiftly and effectively.

Here are descriptions of these common stress complaints and suggestions about how you and your physician may be able to deal with them. Although you have encountered them before in other discussions in this book, I've placed them here to remind you once again of their importance. Also, you should use them as a checklist when you are dealing with bad stress.

"Little" Complaint #1: Chronic Fatigue

As many people experience increasing stress, their energy levels seem to lag. I often hear overworked patients say, "I've

---

just lost my get-up-and-go." Or, "I often run out of steam." Or, "I always seem to feel so tired."

These feelings of fatigue can undercut all motivation to exercise regularly or to carry on the ordinary activities of daily life. But there is no need to give up when you encounter fatigue—as the following solutions demonstrate.

Common solutions.

Many times, something can be done about feelings of fatigue or lassitude. These responses have worked well for patients I know:

• Lower your stress levels.

Fatigue is often a symptom of boredom or stress, and conversely, stress may result from being bored. I always ask my patients how they feel about their work, families, and other aspects of life. If they are unhappy or dissatisfied in some way, excessive fatigue may plague them regularly. In contrast, those who can learn to resolve their stresses and inject more relaxation, excitement, and interest into their lives are rarely tired.

• Increase your level of exercise.

A sense of being run-down or tired all the time may reflect a lack of fitness. People who are in good physical shape naturally feel more energetic.

If you are feeling tired, check your fitness program. Have you been neglecting it? If so, return to your training, and you will most likely find that you perk up, and your energy returns.

• Analyze your diet.

Eating poorly will always introduce the possibility of fatigue. After all, your body needs adequate fuel to function properly. If you are in the habit of skipping meals (including breakfast) or taking in too many "hollow" calories, such as sweets, your energy levels can decline.

Older people may confront special problems because as they age, their appetites may decrease, sometimes because the senses of taste and smell become less sharp. Again, with a loss of appetite, energy levels can decline, and fatigue can enter the picture.

Check your diet and see that you are eating well-balanced meals. Your physician may help you identify certain times during the day when you are especially vulnerable to fatigue. Once again, the culprit could be your diet. For example, if you tend to run out of steam late in the morning or afternoon, you may be running out of calories. To increase your energy at these times, try eating a complex carbohydrate snack, such as an orange, apple, or other piece of fruit.

• Get more sleep.

As we saw in Chapter 3, interrupted sleep or a lack of sleep can cause fatigue in people of any age, but especially in people over forty.

• If fatigue persists, your doctor may be able to uncover physical causes of the problem.

Much has been written lately about chronic fatigue syndrome, which some researchers have linked to deficiencies in the immune system. Also, enzymes produced by the brain, such as monoamine oxidase (MAO), have been tied to chronic fatigue. If your physician determines that there is a biological cause for your lack of vigor, he or she may be able to prescribe medications, such as amphetamines, to counteract the problem.

Our diagnostic abilities for chronic fatigue may soon be enhanced by the use of nuclear medicine techniques. These are currently able to show a difference in tissues in the brains of patients who suffer from chronic fatigue. Eventually, such techniques may enable us to formulate much more effective treatments for fatigue.

"Little" Complaint #2: Back Pain

Perhaps the worst minor complaint for those who want to pursue an active, athletic life is a backache. If you have had one—and the chances are that you have—you know how this ailment can completely stymie your efforts to keep active.

Researchers estimate that up to 90 percent of our population will experience significant pain in the lower back during their lives. Fortunately, these backaches are usually short-lived and have no serious, long-term health consequences. Many of these problems arise from muscle spasms that occur in the lower back during a seemingly innocent movement, such as tying the shoelaces.

On the other hand, nearly half of the population has more serious back ailments. For example, some develop *sciatica,* or pains radiating down the back of the thigh and into the lower leg. This condition usually arises from a slipped or herniated disk in the lower spine or from other problems that damage or put pressure on the sciatic nerve.

Common solutions

The usual remedy for minor backaches is this: Take analgesics, such as aspirin or acetaminophen (Tylenol®). Avoid doing anything that would strain the back for about a week, though staying active and moving about can be helpful.

Warning: You should not try to keep up with your normal, rigorous training routine until your back problem has been resolved. Those who become impatient and try to exercise too soon often reinjure their backs.

More serious backaches, such as sciatica, can often be resolved through rest and more powerful painkilling medications or special rehabilitative exercise programs. In some cases, however, surgery may be required.

How can you *prevent* the onset of back pain? Here are some guidelines:

• Lower your stress levels.

• Avoid unusual, strenuous movements that your fitness training has not prepared you for—even if you did the movements regularly when you were younger.

For example, I know of a man who was an excellent oarsman when he was in college. He continued to keep in shape with vigorous calisthenics and running after he graduated, but he did not pursue specific workouts that would prepare him to row again.

When he was in his late forties, he tried once again to row in the same vigorous fashion as when he was in college. As a result, he developed back and leg pain with sciatica. The unusual strain on his back caused a disk in his spine to slip and put pressure on the sciatic nerve.

The lesson: No matter what your athletic background, before you embark on any rigorous exercise activity, be sure you spend *plenty* of time preparing for that activity, with systematic conditioning exercises.

- Avoid quick, vigorous movements unless you are sure you have warmed up properly.

The warm-up, which should be part of every regular exerciser's training program, is particularly important for older people. I always begin with stretching, including the Williams exercises. These involve lying flat on my back and then pulling up one leg by the knee until the knee almost touches the chest and holding that position for about fifteen seconds. I then repeat the motion with the other knee, and I finally pull up both knees together for another fifteen-second "hold."

When I finish my stretching, I often start my main workout by performing light, careful movements that mimic the more vigorous movements of running. For example, I may walk briskly or jog slowly for about a quarter mile to warm up before I increase my speed during a conditioning run.

- Concentrate on regular exercises that strengthen and condition your back.

All adult exercisers should pay increasing attention to conditioning their backs as they age. Remember, a back injury almost always results from stresses and strains that place unusual pressure on flabby muscles or stiff ligaments and joints. If you keep your back in shape, you will avoid these injuries.

"Little" Complaint #3: Insomnia

Our discussion of sleep and insomnia in Chapter 3 covered many issues on this subject, but some practical observations need extra emphasis.

First, as you age, your sleep patterns will probably change. You may become sleepy earlier in the evening; you may not be able to get to sleep for an hour or more when you go to bed; you may wake up one or more times in the middle of the night; or you may wake up too early and not be able to get back to sleep.

In many cases, these changing sleep habits or needs are just something you must adjust to as you age. You may want to consider these suggestions:

If you become sleepy early in the evening, go to bed! If you wake up earlier than you want, get out of bed and go about your business. If you become sleepy later in the day, take time out for a nap. You can certainly afford it since your early rising has given you a head start on the day, with more time to take care of your various activities and responsibilities.

But aging is not the only cause of insomnia. Other candidates for provoking sleeplessness include the following:

- The effect of certain drugs, such as appetite-suppression drugs, diuretics, or amphetamines.
- Caffeine and alcohol.
- Unresolved worries and anxieties.
- Depression.
- A lack of adequate exercise.
- Sleep apnea, the condition among older people that may cause snoring and considerable difficulty both in sleeping and in breathing. This condition is now being treated more aggressively and successfully by promoting continuous air flow through a nasal catheter or by using a dental splint.
- A need to urinate frequently. This problem is particularly common among people who experience some degree of incontinence, older men who are developing prostate enlargement (hypertrophy), or those taking diuretics.
- Illness, pain, or other health concerns.

Insomnia that is interfering with daily functioning can be both annoying and a serious health concern. Medical researchers have found that getting too little or too much sleep can increase the risk of heart disease and other serious conditions.

So what can you do to overcome your insomnia?

Common solutions

Here is a checklist that may be useful as you tackle your insomnia:

- Use meditative techniques to help you drift off to sleep. (See Chapters 3 and 6 for suggestions.)
- Do not exercise within three hours of the time you expect to go to bed. If you work out vigorously just prior to retiring, your body may still be too active and on edge for you to go to sleep easily. On the other hand, a brisk but not too demanding walk immediately prior to bedtime may help you relax and get to sleep more easily.
- Try to exercise earlier in the day. Aerobic activity is a natural relaxant, in part because of the release during exercise of the morphinelike neurotransmitters called endorphins, which help calm and sedate the mind and body. Increasing the amount of your regular aerobic exercise should help you overcome restlessness at night.

Some people have found their sleep improves after they drink warm milk at bedtime; others may change their mattresses; and still others may experiment with a different type of evening meal, such as one with smaller quantities of food (particularly fats).

If nothing else works and the insomnia is disrupting your life, your doctor may prescribe a sleep medication. But remember that nearly all of these drugs have side effects, and most of them are potentially addictive.

This discussion completes the final step in the Paradox Prescription, Step #7—which involves going in to your personal physician for regular "stress checkups." Next let's look beyond your present health status toward your future prospects. If you can control the bad stress in your life, how long and how well do you think you will live?

CHAPTER 10

The Longevity Paradox

It has taken me most of a lifetime to see that all good things in life—emotional and physical health, spiritual well-being, rewarding relationships, enhanced creativity, material success—can be traced to a simple, fundamental principle, which I call the Longevity Paradox. In a nutshell, this paradox, which is solidly grounded in current medical research, can be expressed this way:

To live long and well, you must live for each moment.

Understanding the Longevity Paradox begins with the recognition that every long and vigorous life is really just a series of shorter "lives." These individual episodes of personal involvement and activity may last only a few months or years. Or if they span a longer period, they typically require only a part of your attention and time. Yet these "little lives" have infinite value, and consequently, they must be nurtured and guarded closely.

For example, one of your little lives may be a family relationship, which could span a lifetime but certainly isn't your whole life: Maintaining it quite well may require only a few hours of close attention each day or week. Another little life may be a friendship, which needs personal contact just one or two times a week or a month. Or you may take on a very important business responsibility or service project that demands an intense daily commitment of your time for a limited period of days or weeks. But after that period, the obligation can be considered finished.

Each of these little lives is limited in scope. But the fundamental message of the Longevity Paradox is that every one of these moments of your existence has a far-reaching, even eternal, dimension and value. The challenge of the paradox is first to identify the limited lives that are absolutely essential. Second, you must discipline yourself to treat each of your indispensable moments with tender loving care.

Of course, as you attempt this balancing act, you will encounter many pitfalls. You may fool yourself into assuming that one of your important little lives is really not *that* important. Or you may become confused about your priorities and lose sight of just how significant a relationship or commitment really is. It's easy to begin to think in these terms:

- *My spiritual life is important, but there will be time for that later.*
  And you end up never making time for the Spirit.

- *My health and fitness are important, but they have to take a backseat right now to my new work schedule.* And exercise never makes it into your life.
- *My child is important, but at least for the short term, I have to give a priority to this social engagement.* Yet you rarely find any time at all for that child.
- *My spouse is important, but I can't restrict my personal freedom.* And freedom soon turns into license.

Obviously, you have to make constant adjustments to accommodate many responsibilities and activities. But major problems arise when you consistently push one essential part of life out of the picture altogether. As brief or limited as your short-term segments of existence may be, you must manage each one well. You must carefully orchestrate each one, so as to fit harmoniously into the whole of life. That's the only way you can expect to maximize your long-term happiness and productivity and maintain the mental and physical balance required to live long and well.

Why the Longevity Paradox Is So Important

The stress of living a life that is out of kilter can take a terrible toll. It doesn't matter whether an important relationship, activity, or responsibility is damaged or destroyed because of neglect or because of a conscious, intentional decision to bow to other pressures or concerns. The final result is the same: The life that is not properly tended and organized from moment to moment is the life that is in danger of becoming "nasty, brutish, and short," as the seventeenth-century British philosopher Thomas Hobbes described the natural, undisciplined human condition.

Furthermore, those who fail to nurture their essential individual moments will often fall prey to the ravages of bad stress—burnout, disease, business failure, or spiritual dryness. Their specific medical problems may include ongoing anxiety, depression, high blood pressure, heart disease, reduced immunity, or a variety of other ills. In the end, such people are likely to die before their time, well short of their potential genetic life span.

That is just the dark side of the stress story. There is another side—the promising Paradox Prescription, my practical program for responding to negative stress. To make full use of the various treatments and suggestions that have been discussed in the foregoing pages, however, you need to keep the more fundamental principle, the Longevity Paradox, in mind. You must confront and overcome bad stress on an hour-by-hour and day-by-day basis. The long and productive life that is possible when bad stress is under control depends entirely on how well you manage the individual moments of life.

By cultivating these moments carefully, you can transform negative stress into positive stress. When that happens, you can begin to speak of enhanced personal power and the possibility of living a longer, more energetic, and more productive life.

I can think of many people who have succeeded to one extent or another in managing their stress by the moment—and dramatically changing their lives and levels of happiness. But in some ways, the epitome of this approach may be a businesswoman whom I'll call Laura.

Laura Discovers the Power of the Paradox

Laura was a patient who was a forty-three-year-old business consultant and mother. Displaying classic signs of burnout, she complained of irregular heartbeats, a frequently upset stomach, stiff muscles, and morning headaches. A physical examination revealed that her blood pressure was higher than it had been during a previous exam about two years before.

It became evident after a lengthy discussion about Laura's personal health habits and life experiences that she was having a severe reaction to the stresses in her life. She was trying to work nine or ten hours a day at her job *and* be a good wife *and* be a perfect mother for her two preadolescent children.

Unfortunately, Laura's husband, who also held down a full-time job, felt that he was too tired when he returned from work to help Laura very much around the home. As a result, Laura shouldered the burden of taking care of the home and family entirely by herself. Arguments with her husband and children had been escalating, and she had been alternating between feeling "numb" and mildly depressed. She was constantly tired and sensed no joy or excitement in her life. Laura was on the verge of an emotional and physical breakdown. She was trying to work too hard, please too many people, and bear too many responsibilities.

Such personal and occupational burnout has been described in the November 1994 issue of the *British Dental Journal* as a syndrome of emotional exhaustion, depersonalization, and reduced personal accomplishment. According to the researchers from the Department of Dental Public Health, London Hospital Medical College, this condition often occurs in individuals whose work involves close personal contact with other people.

This description fit Laura quite well. She was so overloaded in her work and private life that she couldn't seem to squeeze in any opportunity for the simple pleasures she had enjoyed in the past. These included having an occasional lunch or breakfast with close women friends, exercising, and spending a little time each day completely by herself. She couldn't even seem to find a few minutes to pray, meditate, or plan her daily schedule. The lack of time for spiritual reflection was particularly disturbing to her because she placed a high value on her inner life.

The advice I gave Laura was in part medical and in part personal. First of all, I told her that I had been in situations similar to hers at different times in my life. But I emphasized, "I've learned that you can't allow yourself to continue on this track for too long, or you will run completely out of gas."

I noted that we often get the first signals of bad stress from our emotions and relationships. Then, our bodies start saying, "Danger! Danger!" Laura was well into this stage and was swiftly approaching the final, most dangerous zone of stress "illness," where serious impairment of health and relationships may result.

In Laura's case, there was a very real threat that her high blood pressure, heartbeat irregularities, and gastrointestinal problems might become chronic. Furthermore, her deteriorating family situation might easily lead to divorce or a rupture of relationships with her children by the time they entered their teenage years.

"Now is the time to act," I said. "But I would advise you to act by *not* acting—or at least by not acting in the way that you have acted in the past."

Understandably, Laura was puzzled because on the surface, what I had just told her didn't seem to make sense. In effect, I had posed a paradox. After all, the way we usually try to solve problems is to grab hold of them and wrestle them to the ground. Then, we move on to the next challenge—or so the scenario is supposed to go.

Sometimes, when an issue is relatively simple or limited, or we happen to have plenty of time, this aggressive, take-the-bull-by-the-horns approach may work just fine. But too often, our schedules become overloaded, we run out of time to think and plan, and stress overwhelms us. When that happens—as was the case with Laura—an indirect, and perhaps paradoxical, approach is preferable.

Specifically, I advised Laura to try this strategy:

Begin acting counter to common sense on an issue-by-issue and moment-by-moment basis in your life. Specifically, allot time to these three activities, which you now feel you don't have time for:

- First, schedule social get-togethers with female friends at least once a week.

You may think, *I just can't spare the time—my family and my work need me more!* But you will most likely find that your family and work lives improve if you take a break, particularly if you can spend time with supportive people who can help when you run into problems on the job or at home.

- Second, set aside time *every day* for physical activity.

I don't often recommend that a person exercise every day because such frequency isn't necessary for good health and fitness. Also, working out too much can lead to muscular and skeletal injuries.

But Laura needed a consistent, daily break from her other routines. She needed to counter stress at every possible moment. So I placed her on a light stretching and calisthenics program ten to fifteen minutes a day, three times a week. On the other four days, I had her devote at least twenty minutes each day to fast walking.

"And don't tell me you don't have the time for this exercise!" I said. "*Anyone*—including me—can put in some time every day working out. If you develop this habit, you'll find a lot of the stresses you are feeling will begin to disappear."

- Third, I advised Laura to spend some time daily by herself in meditation, quiet reading, or prayer.

"You may have to get up a little early," I advised. "Or you may have to find a quiet corner somewhere during your lunch hour. Or you may just have to disappear for a short time after dinner while the kids are doing their homework. The important thing is to find some private time and space for yourself every single day."

After only a week or two on this new, moment-by-moment, Longevity Paradox routine, Laura found that her life changed completely—and it was a change for the better. Even though she protested at first that she didn't have enough time for these "new" activities, she found—paradoxically—that devoting time to the extra pursuits seemed to give her more time for her family and work. Also, the time she spent on the job and at home was more enjoyable and productive.

Like others who have applied the Paradox Prescription to their stressful lives, Laura stepped back from her problems and, in effect, took a deep breath. Then, she proceeded to tackle her problems by employing a highly unorthodox set of strategies:

- She *spent time on herself*—specifically on personal exercise, relationships, and spiritual development—in order to gain more quality time with her family and at work.
- She *retreated* from her work and responsibilities in order better to fulfill them.
- Though she was under my care and direction as her

physician, she *took the initiative* to collaborate with me as a way of improving her health.

The same kind of success in managing stress is possible for you if you learn to apply the Paradox Prescription in your work and family environments. As you apply these principles on a moment-by-moment basis, you will soon begin to understand the most puzzling, yet powerful, paradox of all:

The negative stress in your life can be transformed into a positive force. It may also become a source of joy as you live longer and better, and experience new surges of energy from the pressures that used to be so oppressive.

In a similar vein, remember these words of the great stress researcher Hans Selye: "Stress is the spice of life. What would life be like if there were no runs, no hits and no errors?"

It is not stress that exhilarates or kills. Rather, your *handling* of stress makes the difference. Stress can help make you successful and happy, or it can ruin your health and well-being. In the end, *you* are the only one who can determine how the stress in your life is to be used, and I trust this book has provided you with some of the guidelines you need to achieve your goals.

INDEX

ABOUT THE AUTHOR

Kenneth H. Cooper, M.D., M.P.H., is the best-selling author of *Aerobics, Controlling Your Cholesterol, Dr. Kenneth H. Cooper's Antioxidant Revolution, Faith-Based Fitness*, and *Advanced Nutritional Therapies*. His books have sold more than thirty million copies worldwide. Dr. Cooper coined the term *aerobics* in 1968 and has received worldwide recognition for his contributions to health and fitness. Dr. Cooper lives with his wife and family in Dallas, Texas.

Improve Your Health with These Other Books
From Dr. Kenneth H. Cooper

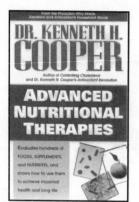

Advanced Nutritional Therapies

A complete guide to untangling and understanding the most recent information on vitamins, minerals, nutrients, and herbs to achieve maximum benefits. Includes a topic-by-topic listing on how nutritional therapy can prevent and heal illnesses and diseases, and improve quality of life.

0-7852-7302-6 • Hardcover • 384 pages
0-7852-7073-6 • Trade Paperback • 420 pages

Dr. Kenneth H. Cooper's Antioxidant Revolution

The bestselling author who helped start the fitness boom with aerobics now offers a powerful program for improved health and well-being. Includes late-breaking research on antioxidants and how they can delay the signs of aging and prevent disease.

0-7852-7525-8 • Trade Paperback • 240 pages

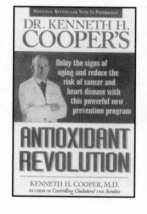

Faith-Based Fitness

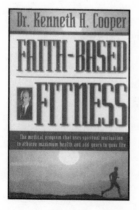

Dr. Kenneth H. Cooper helps you turn your words into action with a comprehensive, on-target regimen that pinpoints the relationship between spiritual faith and physical health. *Faith-Based Fitness* reveals the link between spirituality, and exercise and nutrition that will enable you to live a longer, more energetic life; lower your risks of developing various diseases; handle stress better; experience fewer aches and pains; and more.

0-7852-7137-6 • Trade Paperback • 256 pages